Breast Cancer Recovery: No One Wrote a Manual

The Art of Fran Padgett

Fran Padgett

Book & Cover Design: Cindy Guire, *Ecoveristy*
Printed in India.

Publisher's Cataloging-in-Publication
(Provided by Quality Books, Inc.)

Padgett, Fran.
Breast cancer recovery : no one wrote a manual : the art of Fran Padgett / Fran Padgett.
p. cm.
Includes index.
LCCN 2005926836
ISBN-13: 978-1-886298-18-7
ISBN-10: 1-886298-18-1

1. Padgett, Fran--Health. 2. Breast cancer patients as artists--United States--Exhibitions. 3. Breast cancer patients' writings, American--Exhibitions. 4. Painting, American--21st century--Exhibitions. I. Title.

ND237.P165A4 2005 759.13
QBI05-200118

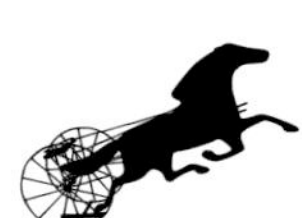

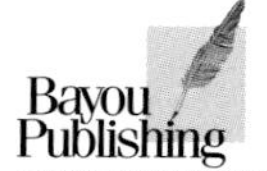

Bayou Publishing, 2524 Nottingham, Houston, TX 77005-1412.
www.bayoupublishing.com (713) 526-4558

This book is dedicated to my mom and to every breast cancer patient of all time.

— *Fran Padgett*

The Road Not Taken

by Robert Lee Frost

Two roads diverged in a yellow wood,
And sorry I could not travel both
And be one traveler, long I stood
And looked down one as far as I could
To where it bent in the undergrowth;

Then took the other, as just as fair
And having perhaps the better claim,
Because it was grassy and wanted wear;
Though as for that, the passing there
Had worn them really about the same,

And both that morning equally lay
In leaves no step had trodden black
Oh, I kept the first for another day!
Yet knowing how way leads on to way,
I doubted if I should ever come back.

I shall be telling this with a sigh
Somewhere ages and ages hence:
Two roads diverged in a wood, and I —
I took the one less traveled by,
And that has made all the difference.

Contents

ACKNOWLEDGMENTS

First, my acknowledgement in friendship and gratitude to my friend, Percy Gentle, a true Texas southern gentleman – "from the old school."

Percy was the first to arrive at the first exhibit of the *Sunrise to Sunrise* paintings, the twelve self-portraits of my body before the mastectomies changed it for all time, the paintings I have called the farewell to my body as I knew it, the paintings of pain.

In slow and deliberate absorption he stopped at each image and each essay. At the last one, he came to where I stood trying to conceal my emotions, and took my hands in his.

"These need to be printed into a book," he told me.

Second, my acknowledgment to a new friend, Sandy Lawrence. Early this year, 2004, the *Moving On* paintings and essays were exhibited. Sandy stopped at each painting and especially at each essay.

She wound her way through the viewers mingling and conversing in surprise and enjoyment, and came to me with a warm hug.

"These are your book," she told me.

Percy, my old friend; Sandy, my new friend, you've convinced me. Here's my book.

— *Fran Padgett*

FOREWORD

There are many ways to react to a diagnosis of breast cancer. Fran's reaction was as creative as the paintings she envisioned and completed.

With her radiant sixth sense ever present and her ingenuity unfurled, she has found herself catapulted into a life more exciting and rewarding than she ever dreamed.

A brave, courageous woman with "a psychic brain and an intuitive heart" as she describes herself, Fran has used the diagnosis as an opportunity to evaluate her life: "How do I want my life to look should the time remaining be limited?"

It is my privilege to know her. I invite you to meet her in the pages of this book.

— *Dr. Joan Weltzien*

PREFACE

These pages present the paintings and "wall stories" from the Houston one-woman art exhibits of my *Sunrise to Sunrise* and *Moving On* series. The essays were written independently of the paintings. The paintings are not illustrations of the essays, nor are the essays meant to provide any further elaboration on the meaning of any individual painting.

I ask you to view each painting and each essay as a vignette, a "snippet of time or emotion" of my life during the first two years of breast cancer.

— *Fran Padgett*

Part I:

Words I never wanted to hear

PROLOGUE

Across the polished wood table my surgeon's face was calm and concerned. His hands were on the open file of pathology reports, his eyes looked directly into mine. I found the sight of his skilled and gentle hands reassuring as I uttered the words that would change my body forever. He had patiently heard my questions and quietly answered them, as I knew he had answered many, many breast cancer patients. But for those few minutes, it was as though I were the only patient in the world to have ever said, "I have decided on the mastectomy option."

"I feel the need to put some things in order," I said, my voice low. "Does it need to be scheduled quickly?"

He assured me that thirty days would have no significant impact on the ultimate outcome. I stood up, shook his hand, smiled, bit my lip, and told him I would see him in exactly 31 days.

My destination: the beaches of Galveston. These chronicles of my breast cancer began in the hours and hours of sleepless solitude facing east across the Gulf of Mexico. Pinks and silver colors of sunrises and flesh flowed from my heart through my hand, filling pages of blank paper.

Next stop: the Gallery. It had been nearly two years since I first heard "invasive carcinoma, 12 o'clock, right breast; 6 o'clock, left breast." My breast cancer chronicles — 32 paintings and 26 essays — were arranged and spotlighted on the gallery walls, to be viewed by family, friends and strangers. In the subdued light, background music mingled with their lowered voices as they stopped in front of each page and each painting. When they turned to me I saw their tears. Yes, my friends, my images and words reveal my heart and bare my soul. Thank you for coming. I love you.

— *Fran Padgett*

Breaking the news… "revolting development"… bullet-proof and dodging a bullet…

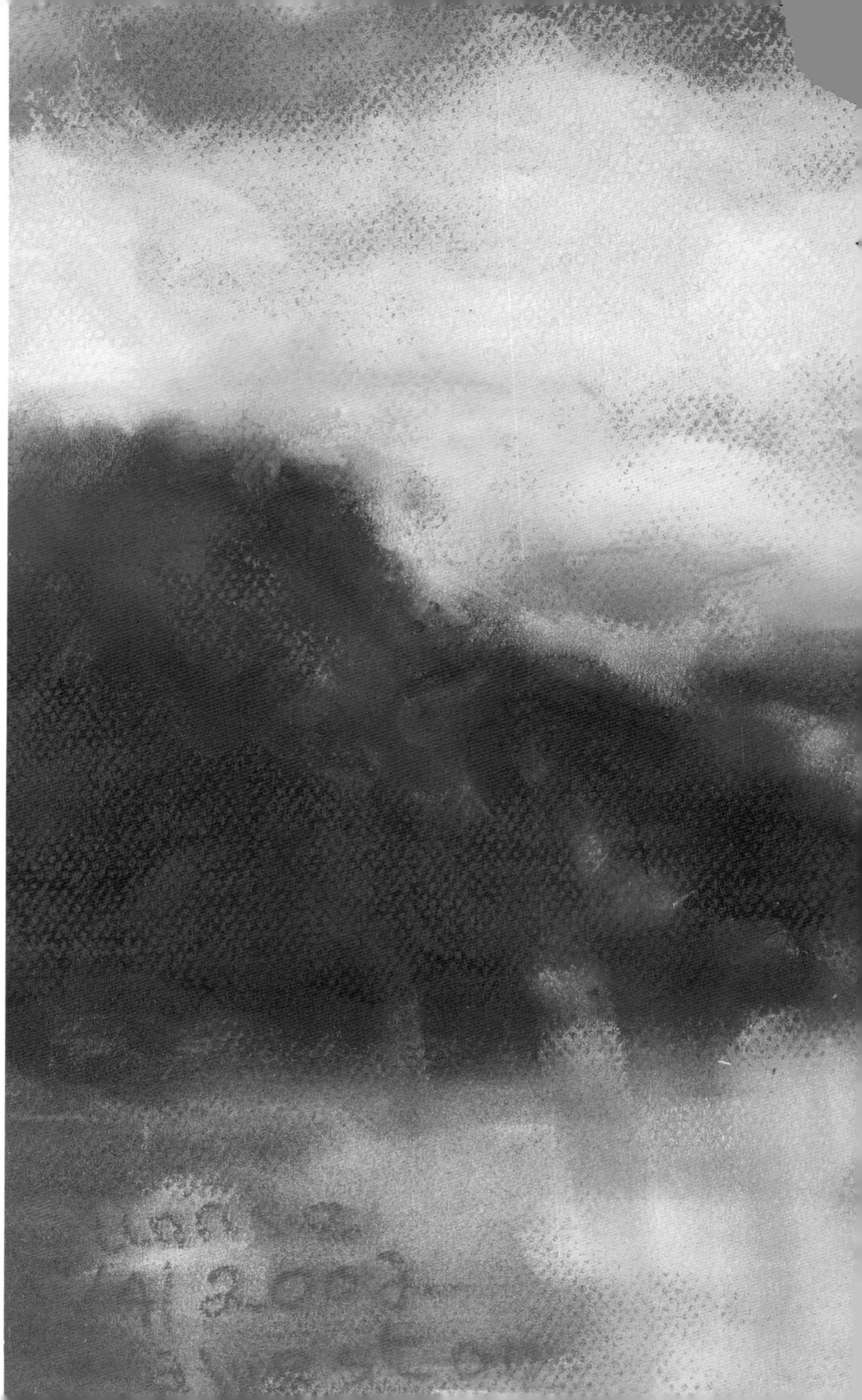

Sunrise I

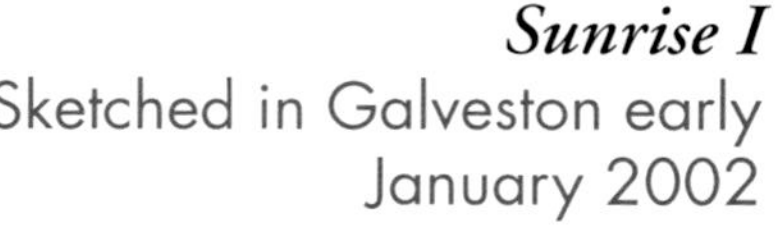

Sketched in Galveston early January 2002

The low-lying bank of clouds obliterated the horizon and the lingering darkness obscured the shoreline, melding the sky and the water and the land.

Evening, early December 2001; on the phone message recorder, Dr. Marlowe's calm voice. "Mrs. Padgett, I have your path report. Please call me back and we will discuss it."

[Well, Dr. M., surely you know that I know that when the path report is uneventful, then Nola calls me…not you.]

Early AM, early December 2001; Mom's voice. "You are calling pretty early, hope nothing is wrong down there." "Actually, Mom, there is a revolting development…I have cancer in my right breast…Incredible…I had always considered myself bullet-proof when it comes to cancer since there is none in our family."

Mom: "Well, darn it."

[My mom is wonderful, and "darn it" was the perfect response.]

Evening, early April 2002; on the phone message recorder, Dr. Marlowe's calm voice. "Mrs. Padgett, I have your path report. Please call me back and we will discuss it."

[Deja vu. My intuition was accurate.]

Dr. Marlowe: "There was ductal and also an invasive lobular…very small, very early. I am so glad that I did not try to talk you out of the left mastectomy…we have certainly dodged a bullet."

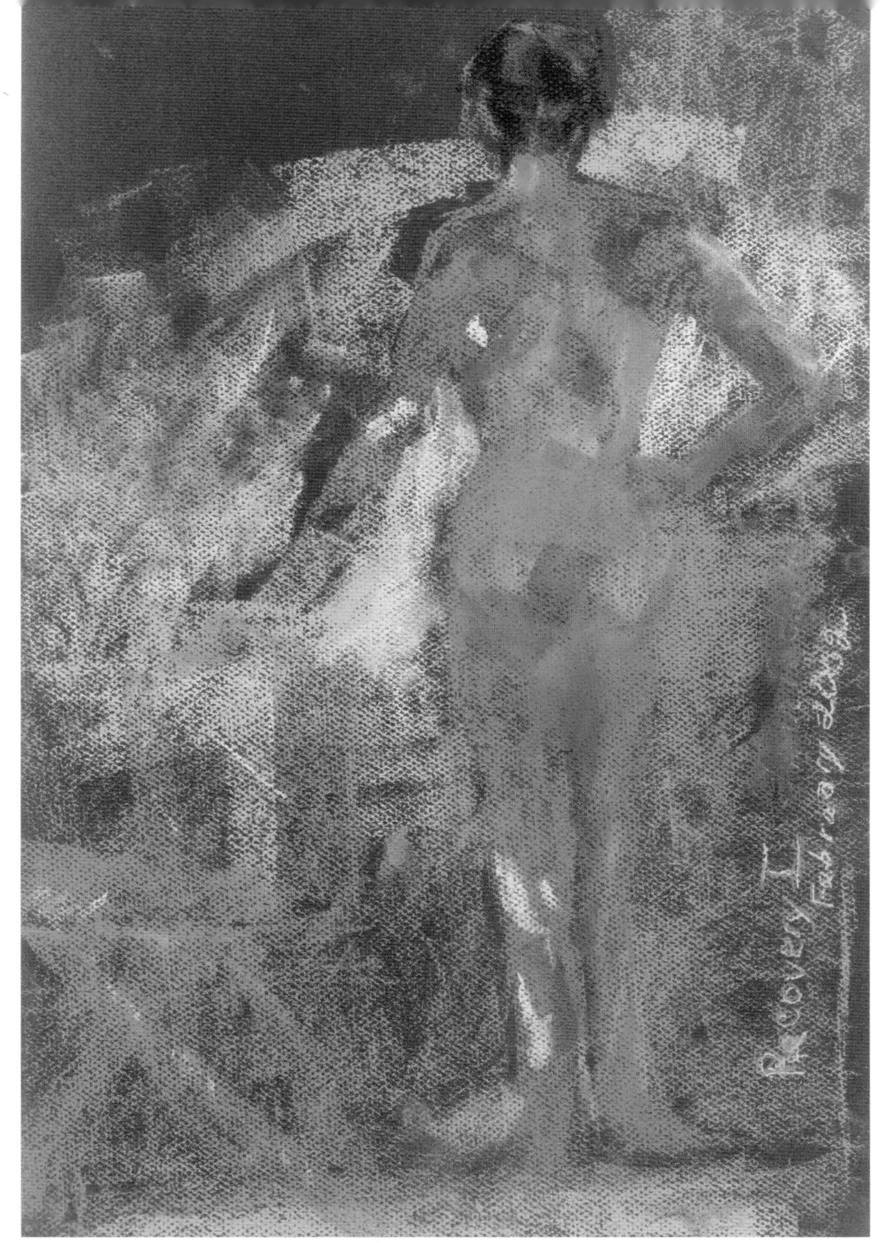

Recovery I

Caught Unaware

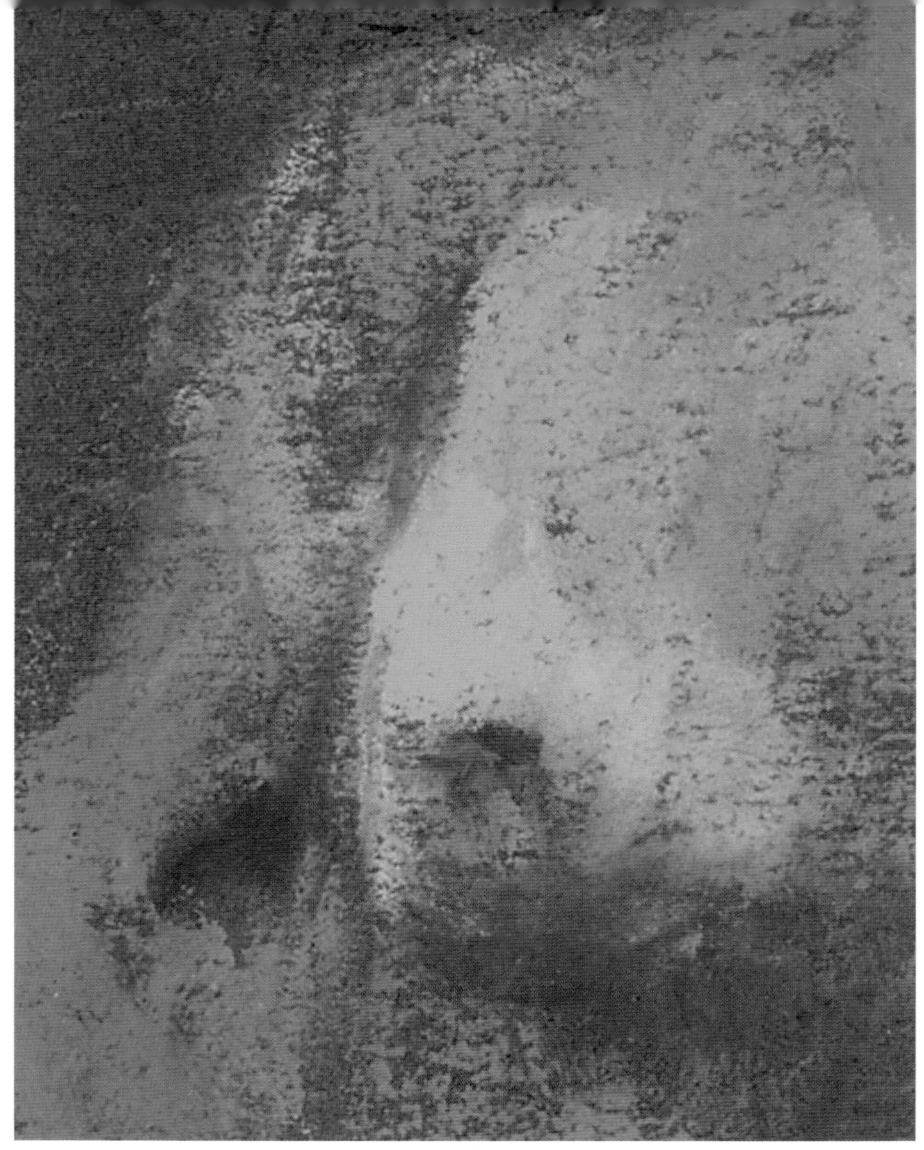

Recovery II

Dammit

Defiance!

Fury!!!

Fear!

Deciding on breast reconstruction, White lies and a wild man ...

Consultation with a magician also known as plastic surgeon, a.k.a. Dr. Haven:

Dr. H.: "Are you healthy?"

"Yes." *[Incredibly accurate, until Dr. Marlowe's phone call.]*

"Do you drink?"

"No." *[Just a little white lie..., champagne doesn't count, does it?]*

"Do you smoke?"

"No." *[Oh well, one white lie leads to another...does it count that champagne calls for small, sweet cigars?]*

"Do you chase wild men?"

"No." *[Actually I would if I could find one!!!]*

Arriving by mail shortly from my Washington D.C. journalist cousin, Carol, a photo-art card of gorgeous-body naked man on white horse *[Lord Godiva?]* "Here's a wild man for you," she wrote. It is still in my purse, like the prince with glass slipper. Someday I may find the wild man who fits.

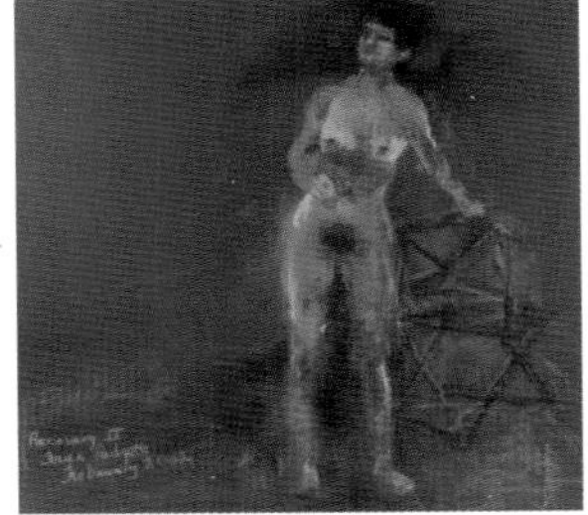

Breast Reconstruction

[Art and skill and wondrous modern materials come together to imitate life]

Dr. Haven: "How voluptuous do you want to be?"

[Wow! Every girl's dream. Do you mean I get to decide that?]

Later…looking down at the imitation breasts (created by "expanders" with scars across them like an equator across the globe…"Dr. H., I didn't think I was really going to be quite so big."

Dr. H.: "We need to make you quite voluptuous."

"Doctor Haven, who in the world have you been talking to?"

[I am learning that voluptuous is one of Dr. Haven's favorite words.]

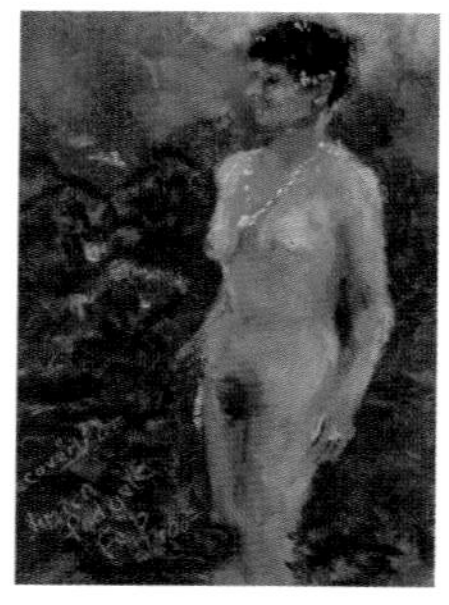

Recovery III
My Camellias (Bloom in December)
Thank you, Mary Jane, my spirited sister-in-law for the kindest favor I've ever been given.

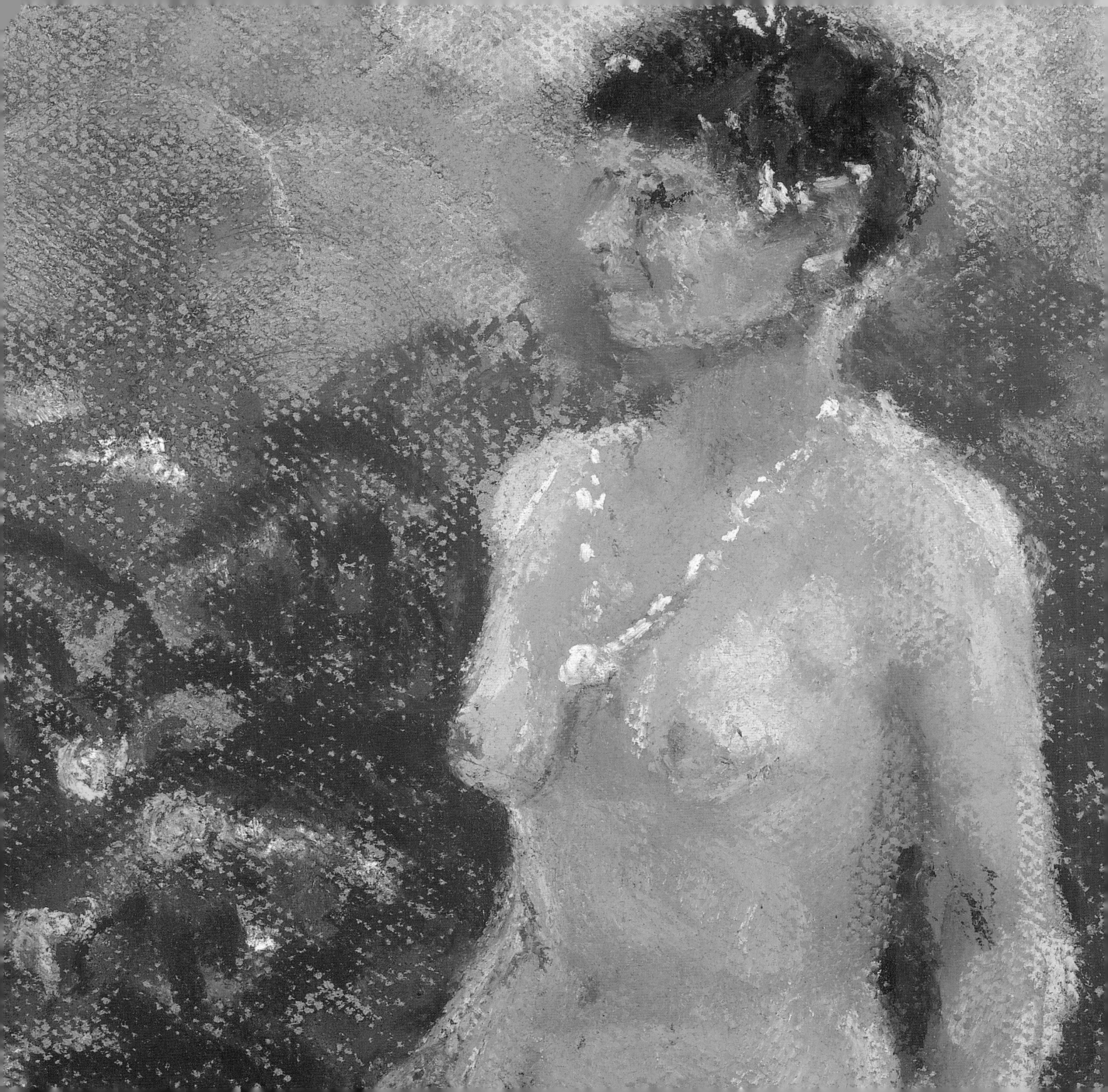

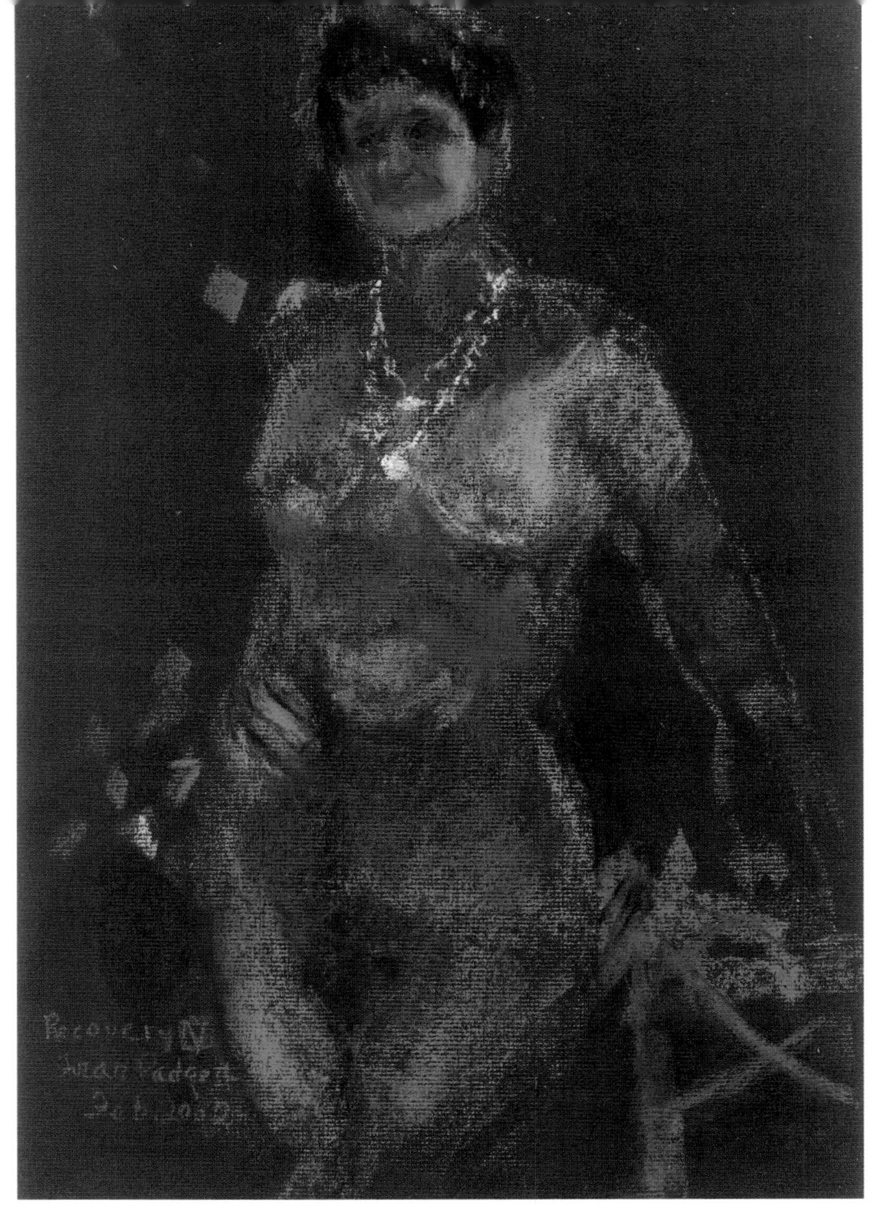

Recovery IV

The Silver Chains

What price glamour?

Drawbacks...

Let's see if I can keep all this straight...my imitation breasts are silicone and my imitation nails are acrylic...or is it the other way around? Wondrous materials. Mostly an improvement over what Mother Nature originally provided, with only a few drawbacks.

"Really, Dane, I could have drowned." (To ease my stress I had been handed some brandy while relaxing in the warm and bubbly waters of the swim-spa.)

"You can't drown in a swim-spa. The water isn't deep enough."

"No, really, I could have. My imitation breasts are NOT flotation devices!"

"Well, they should have been made from Styrofoam."

"I'll make that suggestion."

"I could carve you some."

[What do you know! A wannabe sculptor.]

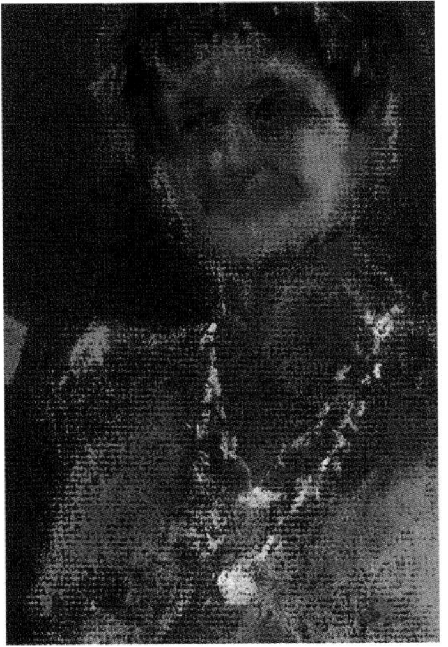

"Every girl's dream!"

"Stacy," I said to my dear and wonderful 13-year old granddaughter. "I am going to have my left breast removed. THEN I will have a 'Barbie doll bustline' all the way across."

Impish grin and sparkling eyes, with instant response:

"Every girl's dream!"

Recovery V
The Dark Window
Reflecting...reflections...hope...and hope...and hope.

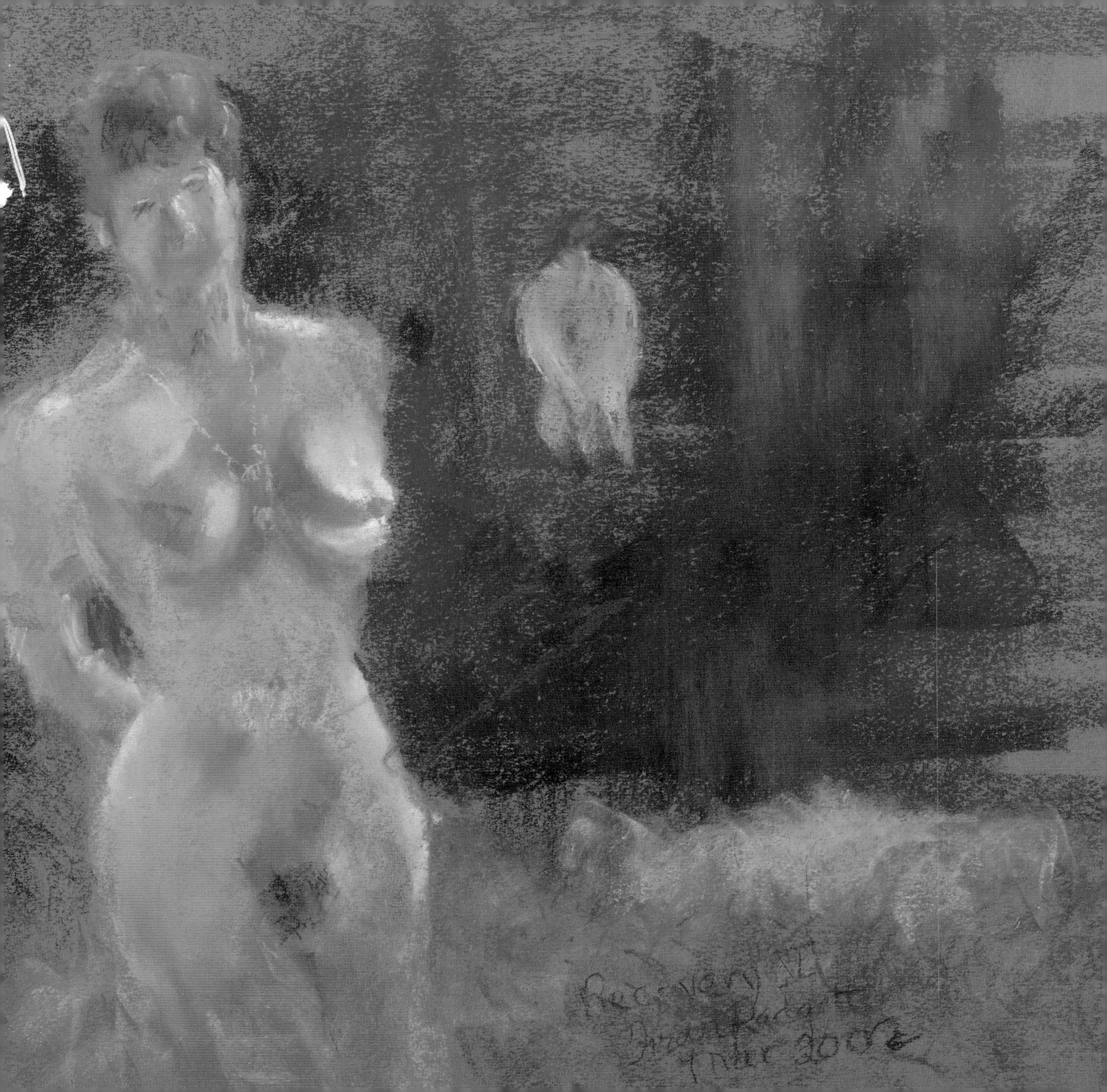

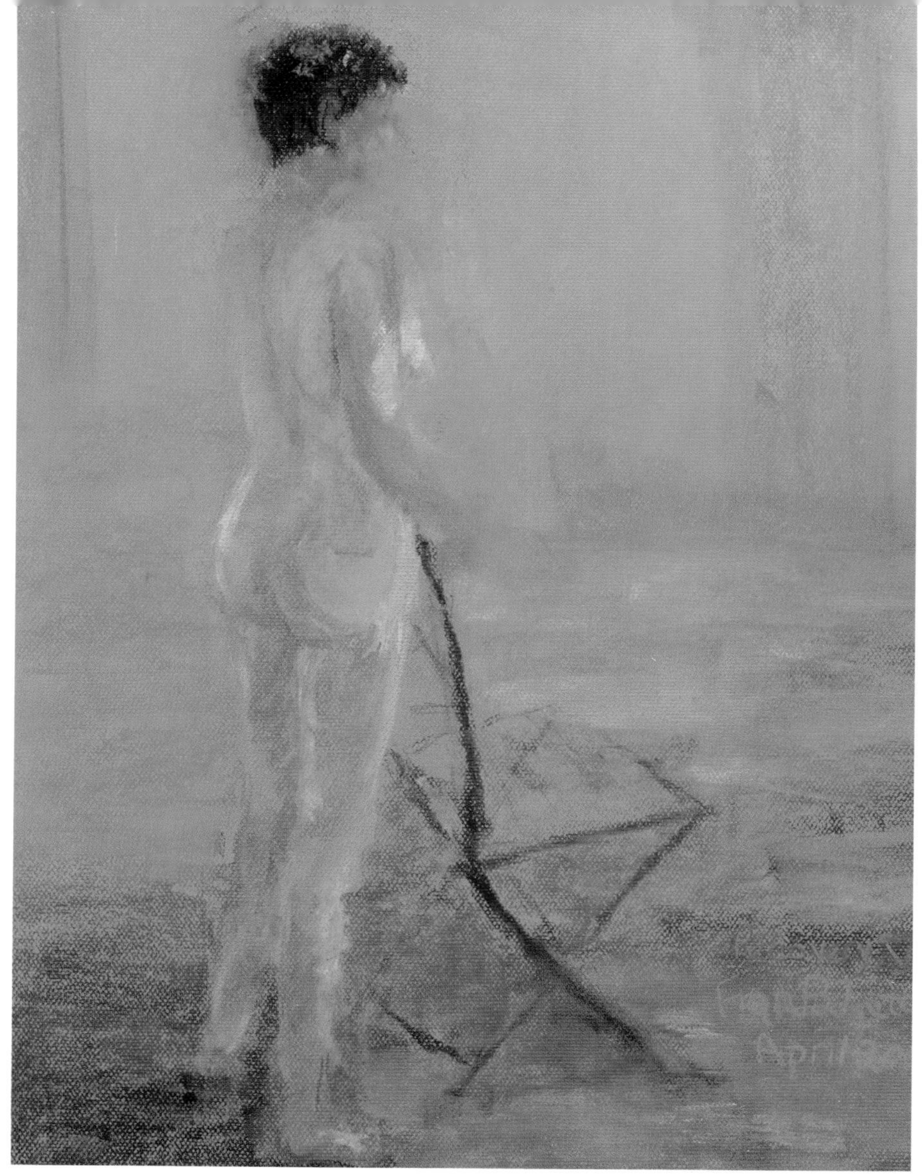

Recovery VI

Facing the Garden Fence

Feeling cornered.
Feeling trapped.

Breast reconstruction starts on the "deja vu" side...

At the end of second or third visit to the magician (Dr. H.) for another injection of saline with a horse-vet sized hypodermic, he turns to make a note in the chart and says,

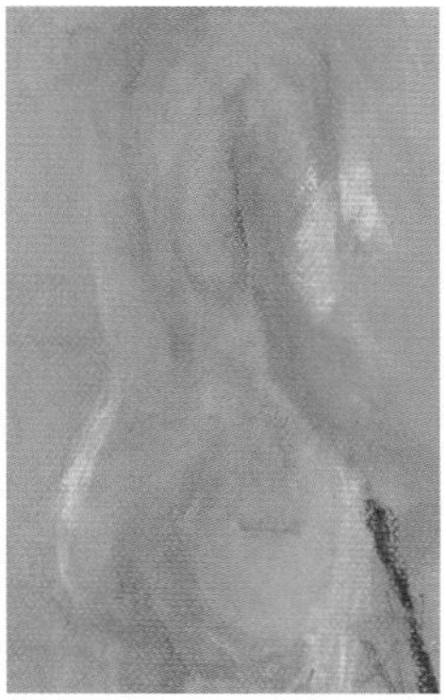

"Fran, you are weird." *[Believe it or not, I have been told that before.]*

"Why?"

"The expander has rotated 180 degrees."

"How can that happen? I don't think I did anything to it."

Dr. Haven likes to joke and tease, I have learned. "Well, maybe it was your boyfriend."

[Yeah, right. One thing I do know...it wasn't the wild man. I haven't found him yet.]

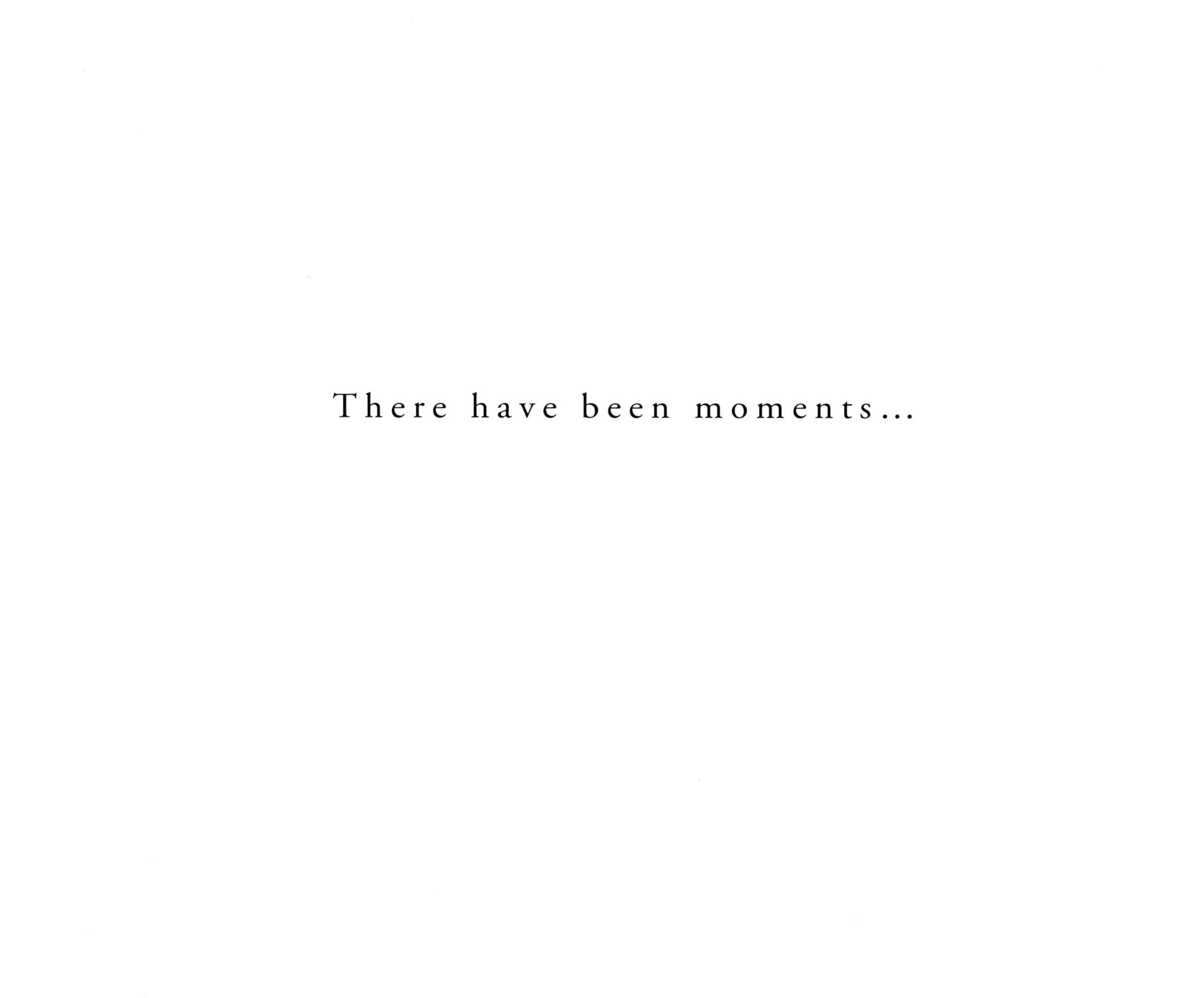

There have been moments...

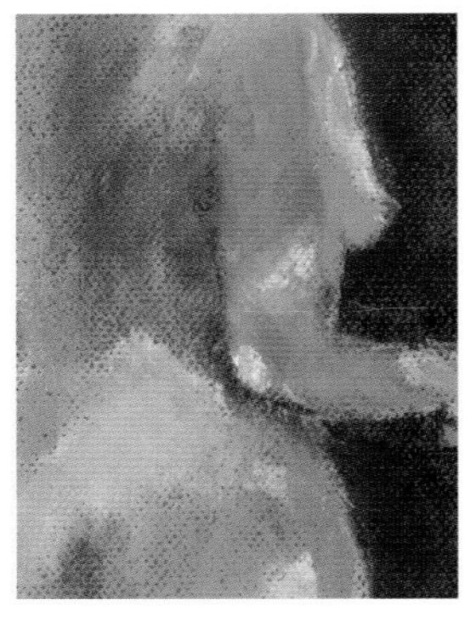

"Leah," I said, "I'm having a hard time deciding if I can go on. I just can't see that it matters if I live."

And Leah, dropping her usual technique of asking gentle, probing questions that cause one to think long and hard and deep, said:

"YES, IT MATTERS IF YOU LIVE!"

"And, this is what you need to do. You have spent all these many, many years living and doing for everyone else. *[True, doesn't everyone?]* And now you have to make yourself the focus of your life. Find something to do that you have a passion for, something that is intellectually challenging to you."

[Leah, you were so right. It took all of three hours for your advice to soak in and realize there are passions.]

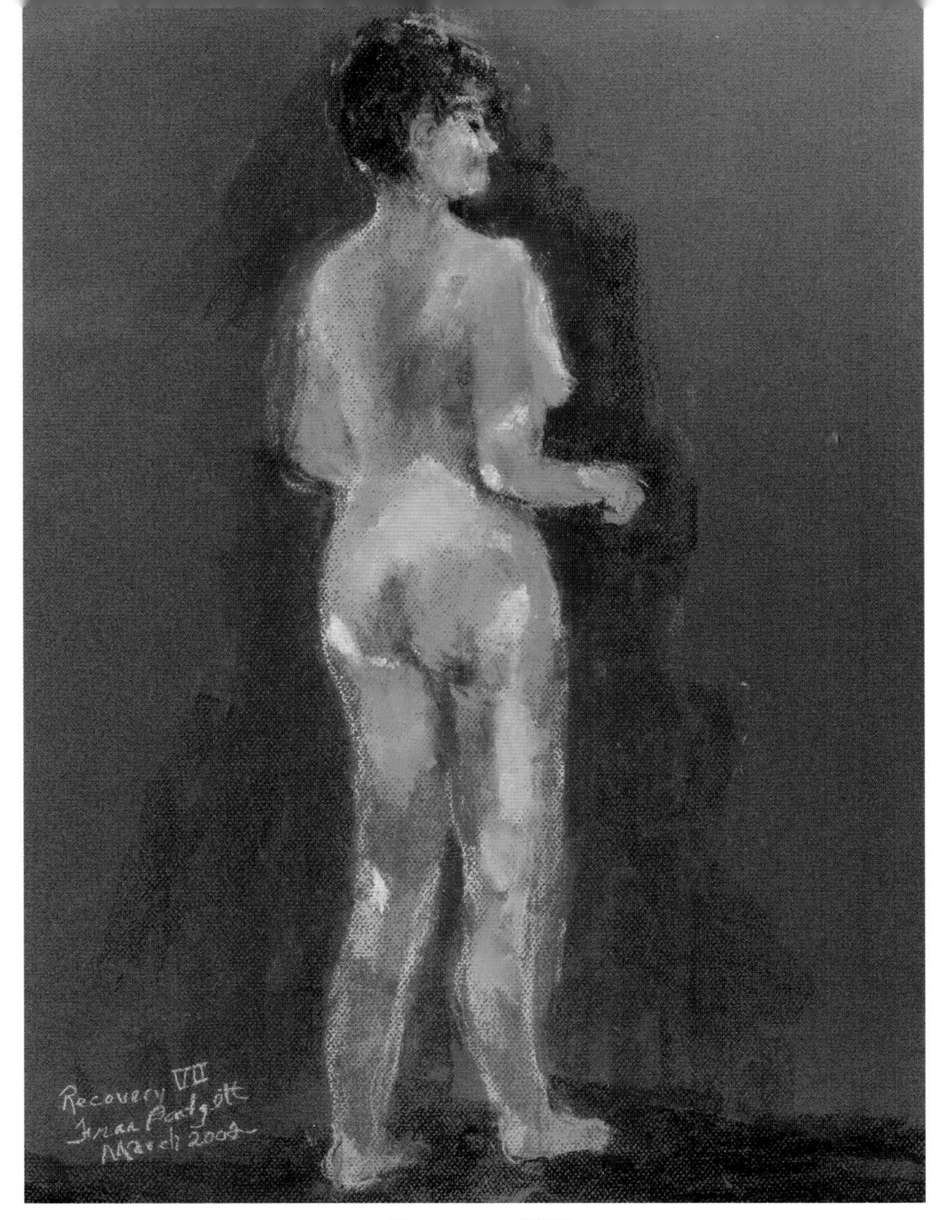

Recovery VII

Bright Sun but No Warmth

And then what price happiness?

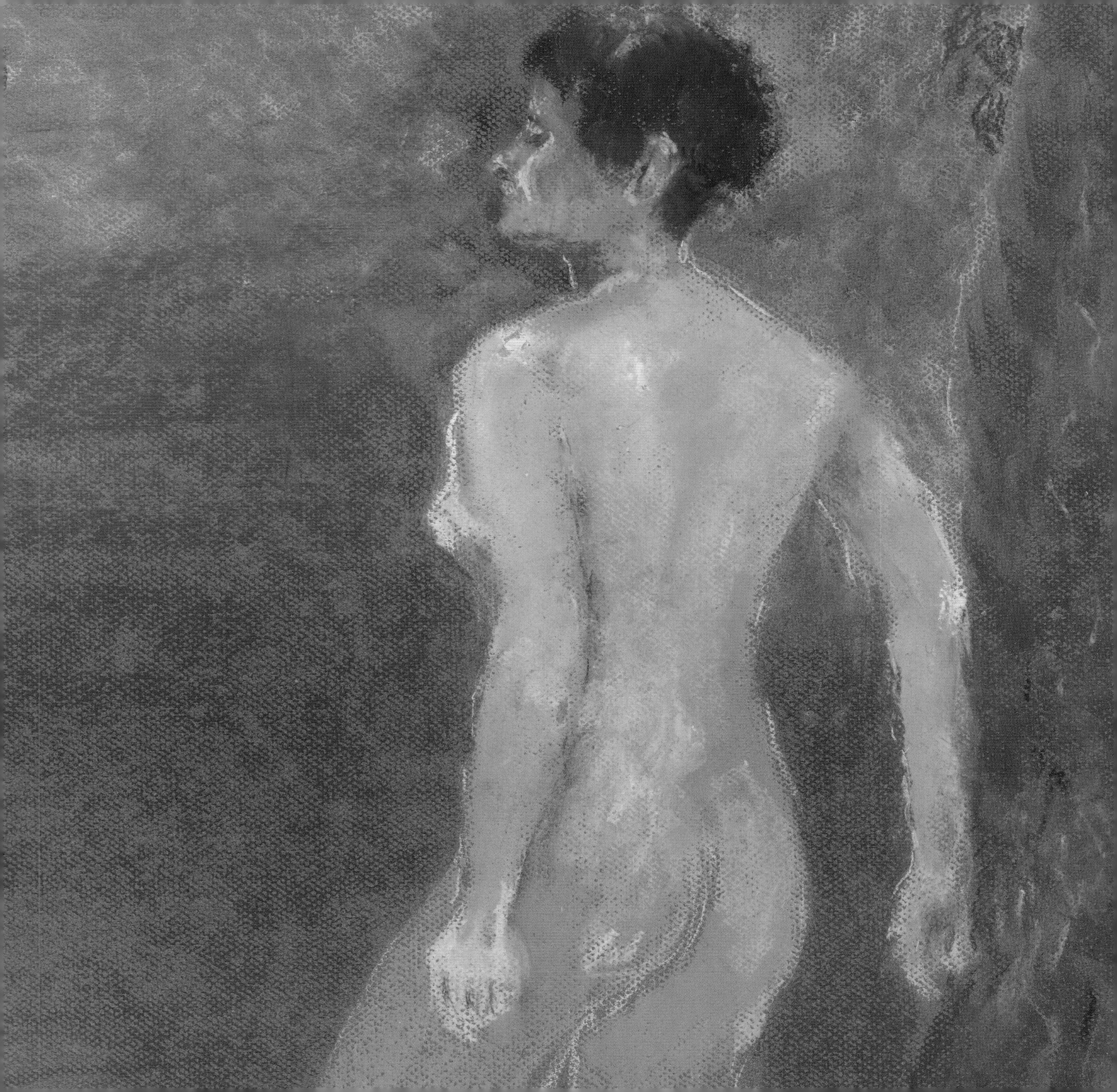

And more moments...

Driving away from an afternoon spent selecting mats and framing materials for these paintings, I am overcome. It has been days and weeks since I have looked at them. Why are there tears now?

And different moments...

The down feeling persists until the next afternoon in the Kroger parking lot. I have put the wine and the flowers in the back seat and get behind the wheel.

A tall, handsome man with dark hair knocks on the car window on the passenger side. He has papers in his hand. Thinking I have left something in the store, I lower the window.

"YOU ARE SEXY," he says. Incredulous, I just wave a dismissing hand at him.

"I mean it," he says. "Is there any chance I could have your phone number?"

Doubly incredulous, I mutter something like "not a chance." He straightens up and walks away.

About a block away, headed home, my palm smacks forehead. "Damn, Fran," aloud to myself, "you could have asked him for his phone number! He could have been the wild man; now you will never know!"

Recovery VIII
Don't Touch Me!
Feelings? A little afraid...and a whole helluva lot angry.

To live the passions...

Two of the passions (the kids and the horses) are expensive, hopefully the third passion can fit in with the first two...

Reconfiguring assets...

Some people speak with a brogue, some with a drawl, some with a twang. People from Washington D.C., like my cousin Carol, are prone to "government-speak."

"Fran," she said, "to make your income you can reconfigure your assets."

"Carol, what in the world does that mean?"

[Reconfigure your assets...hmmmmmmmmmmmmmm...sounds like another way to say breast reconstruction. This is great. Already silicone and acrylic and Styrofoam are getting mixed up in my mind...now I need to keep straight 'reconfiguring' and 'reconstructing'.]

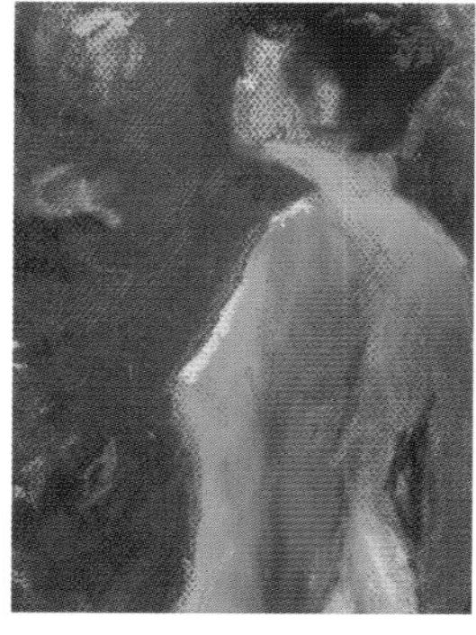

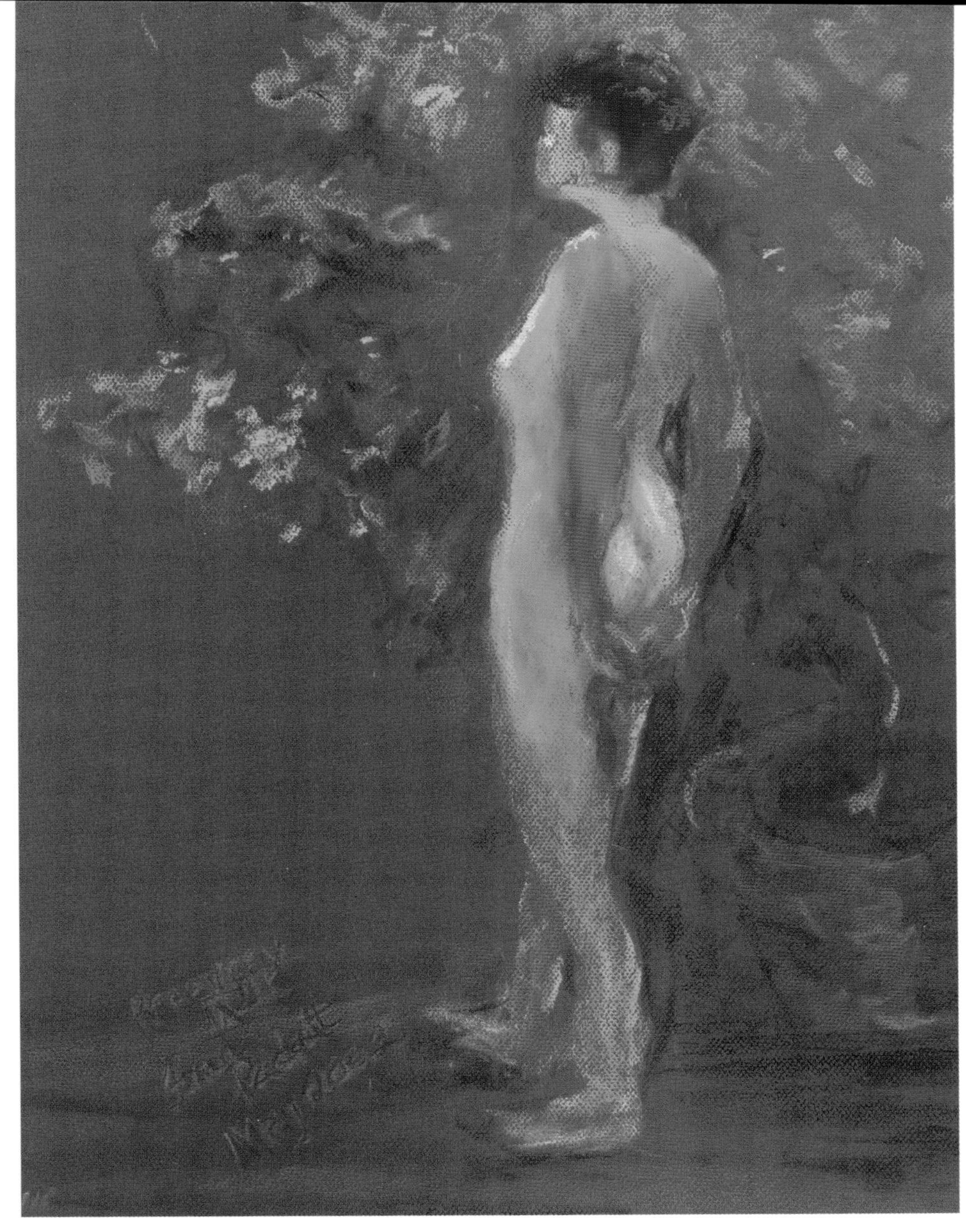

Recovery IX

The Old Ficus Tree

I choose to not dwell on the pain and the fear.

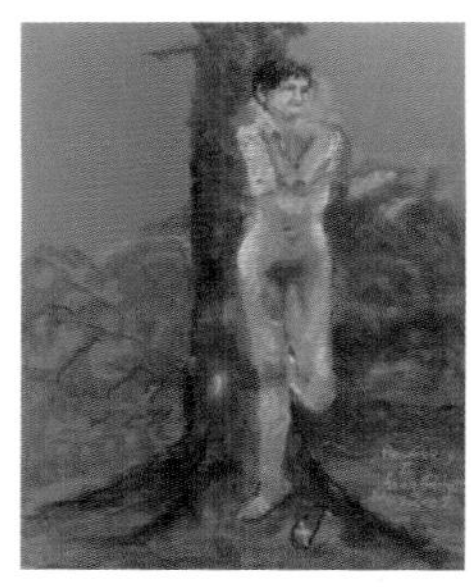

The "A-Team"...

(I wish there were better words than "thank you".)

Phone conversation with Mrs. Simms, the sweet and friendly lady with Cancer Interaction Group (Dialog):

"Your surgeon was Dr. Marlowe? He is great! Who was your plastic surgeon?" she asked.

"Dr. Haven."

"Really! Dr. Haven did my face lift. You had the two best."

"Yes, I believe I did. I have called them the A-team."

THANK YOU, Dr. Haven...for my new 'Barbie doll' bustline...it really does look quite natural, finally *[I did have doubts about it along the way]*...and for my face lift. You said it would be something fun. Maybe I am one of your better works of art.

THANK YOU, Dr. Marlowe... for believing that medicine is ART and science...for knowing that quality of life is paramount even if life is shortened... for listening to and believing in your patient.

Why this exhibit of obviously very personal, emotional paintings by an extremely private person?

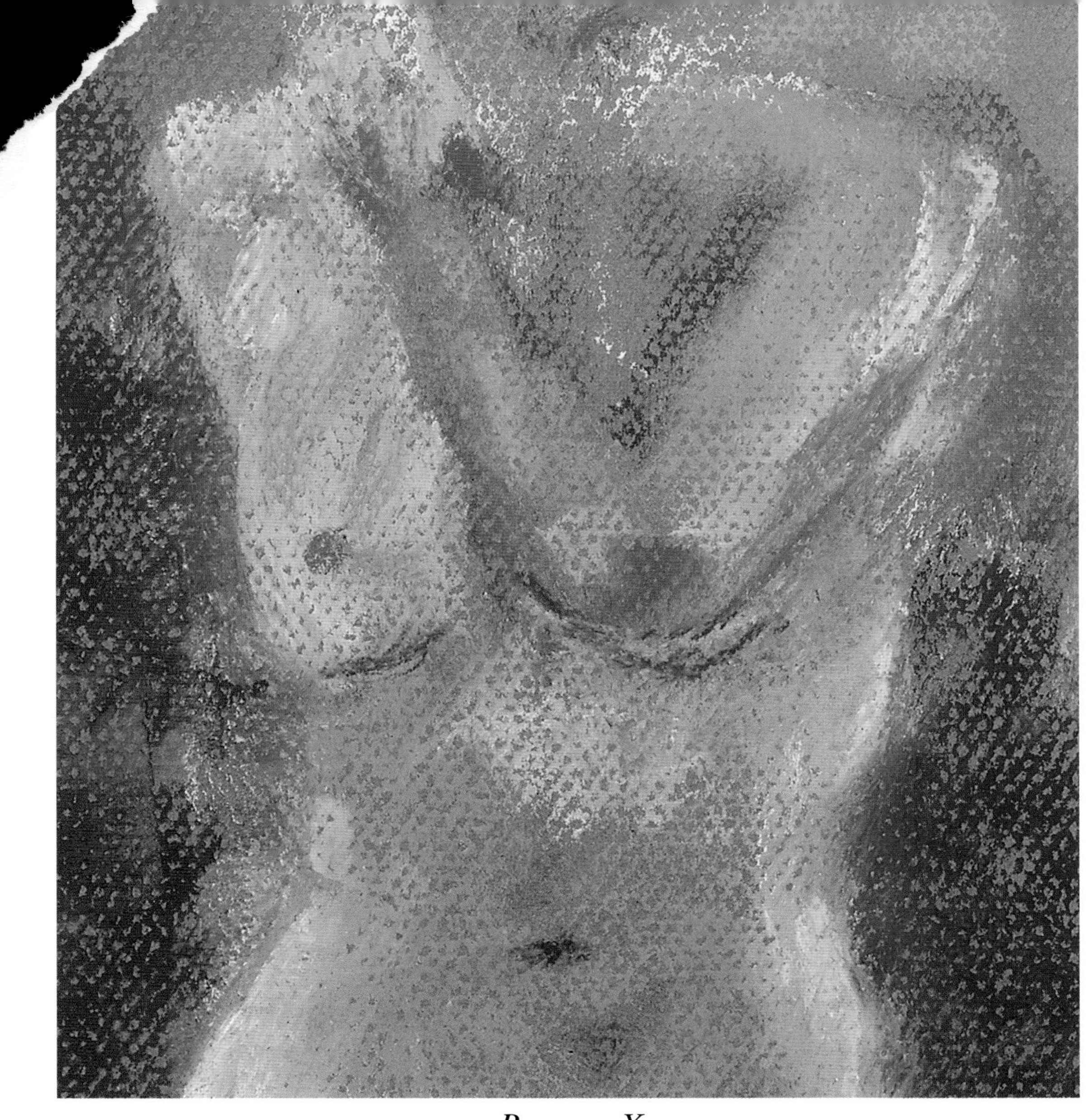

Recovery X

The Tallow Tree

"I conceal my pain; I control my tears."

Cancer is not the scary word it used to be

...or is it?

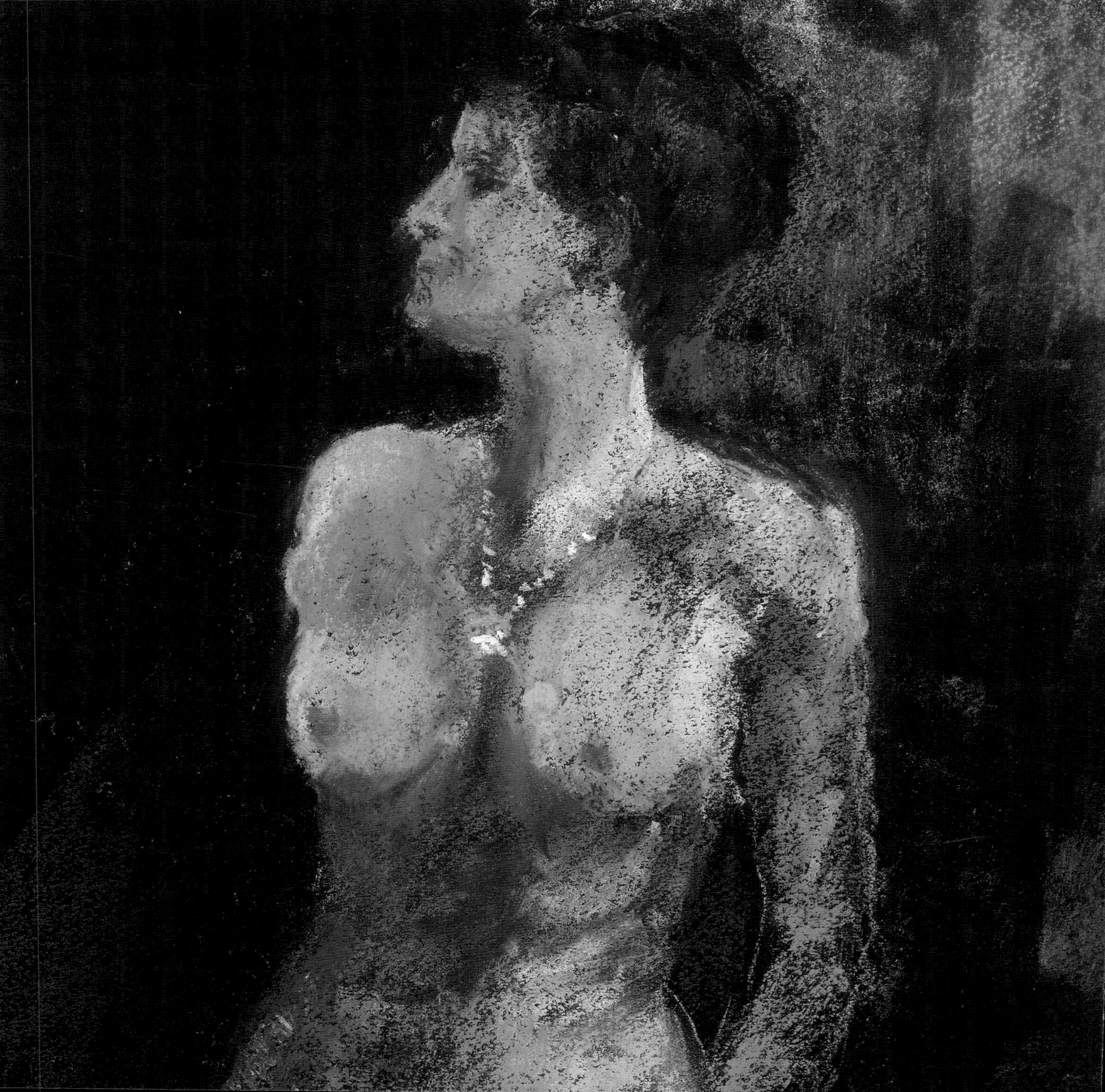

“Why haven’t you told your daddy?”

That question came to me from Karen, the nurse who has helped us take care of my invalid father for 15 years.

“Because, Karen, he would instantly think I was dying. And he would lie there in that nursing home bed and cry. And I would not be able to reassure him enough that I am about to be fine. The last of my surgeries will be soon and when I have pretty much recovered and I can drive up there and walk in and let him hear my voice and smile, and feel my hand and kiss, and see me out of nearly blind eyes, then maybe I’ll tell him…but then again maybe I won’t…because by then it will not matter, will it? If he dies without knowing I have/had breast cancer, then that will have to be for the best.”

Early morning, August 28, 2002, a call from Marlene, the nurse at Arkansas Nursing Center. “You probably want to come today.”

“Marlene, would you hold Dad’s phone to his ear so I can sing to him?” Over and over I sing “Show Me The Way to Go Home” and over and over I reassure him, “Rest easy, Dad. We are going to put you beside your Gramma.” And I hear his breathing change. “He heard you,” Marlene says.

Two hours up the road, Marlene calls. “I’m sorry, Fran. Your Dad has just expired. He was quite a fellow!”

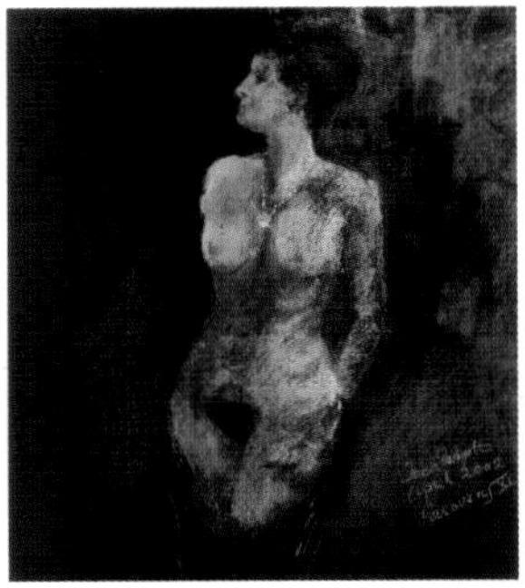

Recovery XI
The Gold Charm
In solitude, strength is found.

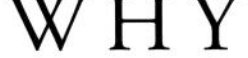
WHY?

For Breast Cancer Awareness Month….the paintings and the conversations being shared are offered in the hopes of conveying encouragement…

…to encourage frequent and timely checkups…early detection (and mastectomies) has meant for me no lymph node involvement, no chemo and no radiation…for which I am exceedingly grateful…

…to encourage the recognition of your passions and then to live one's life with passion.

And for my dear friends both old and new…for my family both near and far away… colleagues, doctors, nurses, Leah (my psychologist), viewers and readers…*my gratitude…there are no words to adequately express.*

Recovery XII
Seated
Ductal. Lobular. Mixed pattern. Pagetoid. In situ.
More than I ever wanted to know.

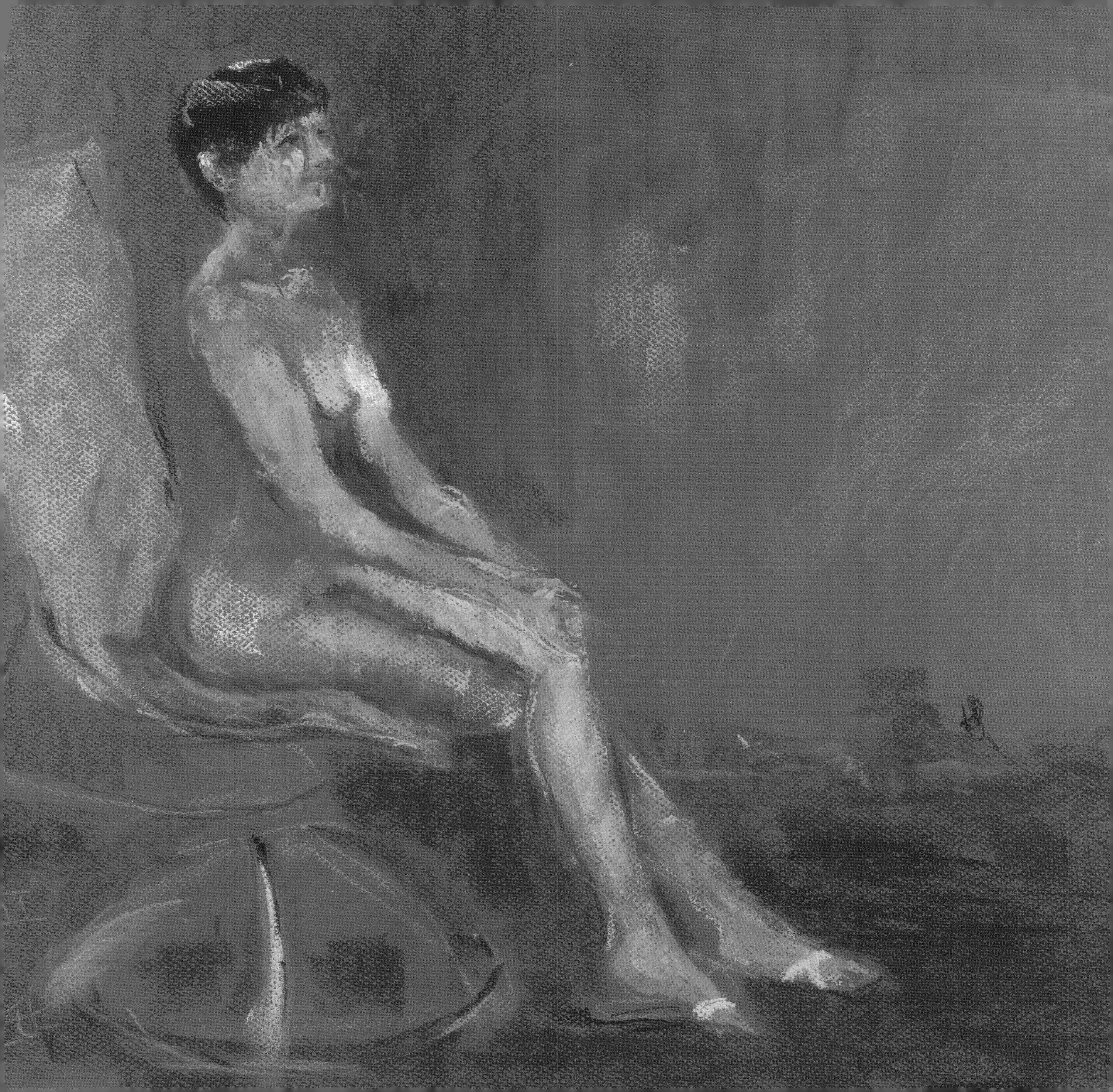

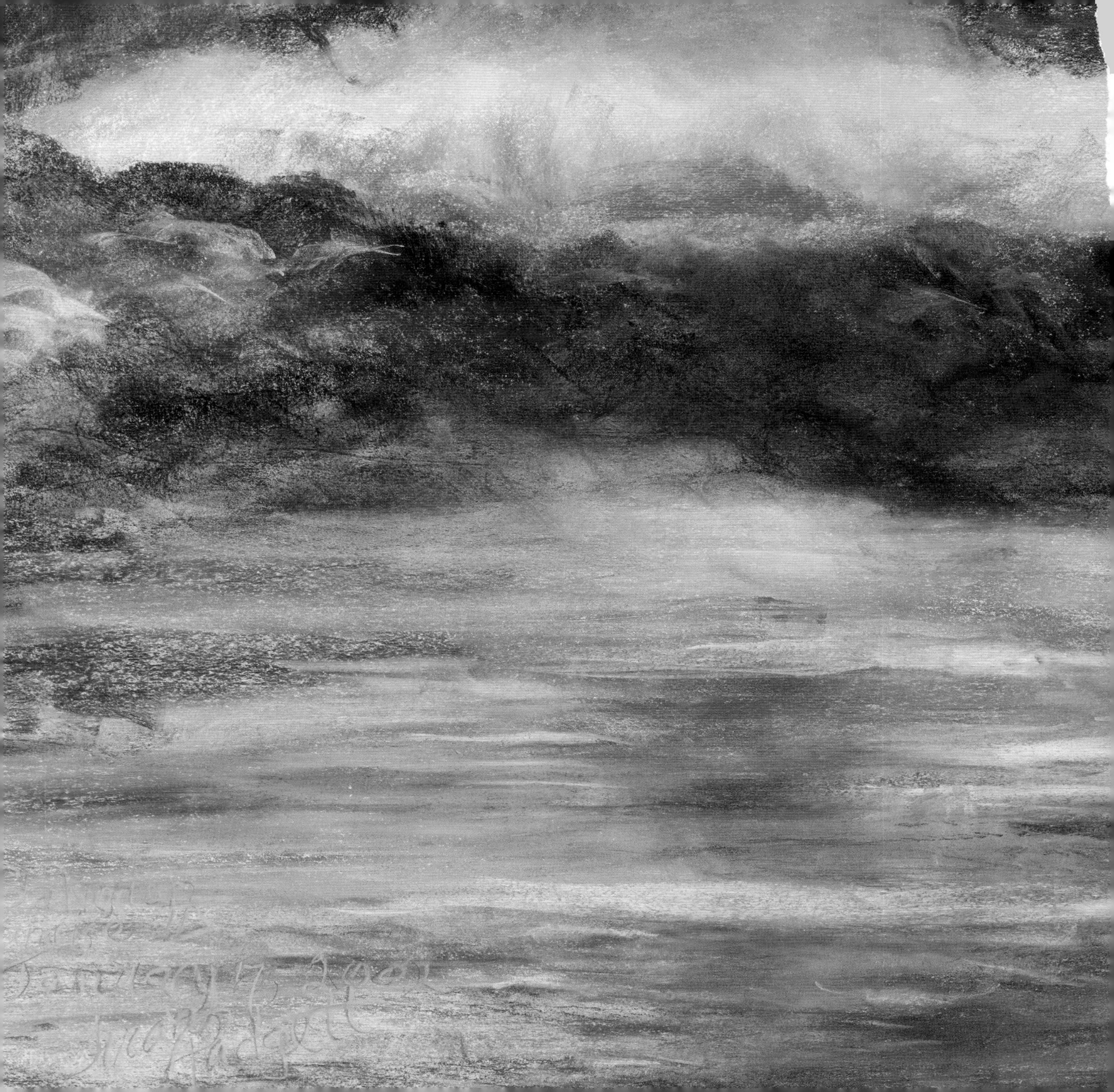

Sunrise II
Galveston early January 2002.
Solitude…searching…soothing…strengthening

Part II:

Past Recovery, Beyond Reconstruction, and on to *What Makes a Woman a Woman?*

PROLOGUE

Saturday morning, twenty years ago. I walk slowly into the kitchen, stop at the counter beside the sink. "Why do I feel so awful?" I wonder. I cross my arms on the countertop and lay my head on them. It's a good thing I don't have to go the office today, I think to myself. My whole body feels leaden, my mind as lethargic as my body, even though I have had extra sleep, proper food and vitamins, not to mention my usual large cups of morning coffee. Where is my energy? Why can't I think?

I call my mom. Whatever would we do without Dr. Moms? I describe to her the physical and mental inertia I have been experiencing.

"You probably need estrogen," she says. "I know that for me it is my energy."

Dr. Mom, right again!! Like magic, "hormone replacement therapy" lifted me back to vitality.

2002: Breast cancer recovery, early stages. Houseguests are visiting us for a weekend. I leave them talking at the dinner table, walk into my closet and curl up on the floor in the fetal position. My mind is virtually blank. "I don't want to see anyone," I confide to my husband, who has found me huddling in the dark. Shortly he returns with that little yellow tablet. "Take it," he says gently.

He knew.

Four months: no estrogen.

Four days: Tamoxifen.

Gott en himmel!! I can't live like this. I have to be ME.

I sit across the polished wood table from Dr. Marlowe. As always, he is calm, and as always, patiently listens.

"Hot flashes, yes, but I can deal with those. Night sweats, yes, but I can stand that." I pause to gain control. "But I can't face life not feeling like ME. It is estrogen that makes me feel good. It is estrogen that gives me energy. And more than that," I tap my forefinger on my forehead for emphasis, "I need it to be able to THINK. I have to work, I have to support myself, but above all else I HAVE TO THINK."

He nods slowly, acknowledging that he understands.

"If taking estrogen shortens my life, THEN I TAKE THAT RISK!"

He assures me "We will do whatever it takes to make you feel better." He signs the small square paper with the magic word scrawled on it...that word that means Woman, that means Life, that means Vitality. With tears of relief, I thank him, and leave clutching the prescription in my hand.

And so began the gradual climb back to my creativity, my sanity, myself.

—Fran Padgett

Reconstructed I
(as I am now")
Jan. 2003
[illegible] Padgett

Reconstruction I

Blue Torso and an Angel

Thank you, my friends, for sending good thoughts on wings, making "angel kisses" on my cheek.

One helluva year.

The year was 2002. I call it "ground zero."

Early one morning, mid-January after the first mastectomy, I was still in bed, half awake, and with my eyes closed came the vision of my lop-sided chest.

Before I knew that there would be a second mastectomy and second cancer diagnosis, that my father would not live through the rest of the year, and that I would sadly decide to separate from my husband of many years because I would need to live alone, words came into my head like a psychic prediction: ***Double mastectomy, death, and divorce: This is going to be one helluva year. Will I be up to it?***

Reconstruction VII
Diptych
Leaving you divides us, but you are the larger part.

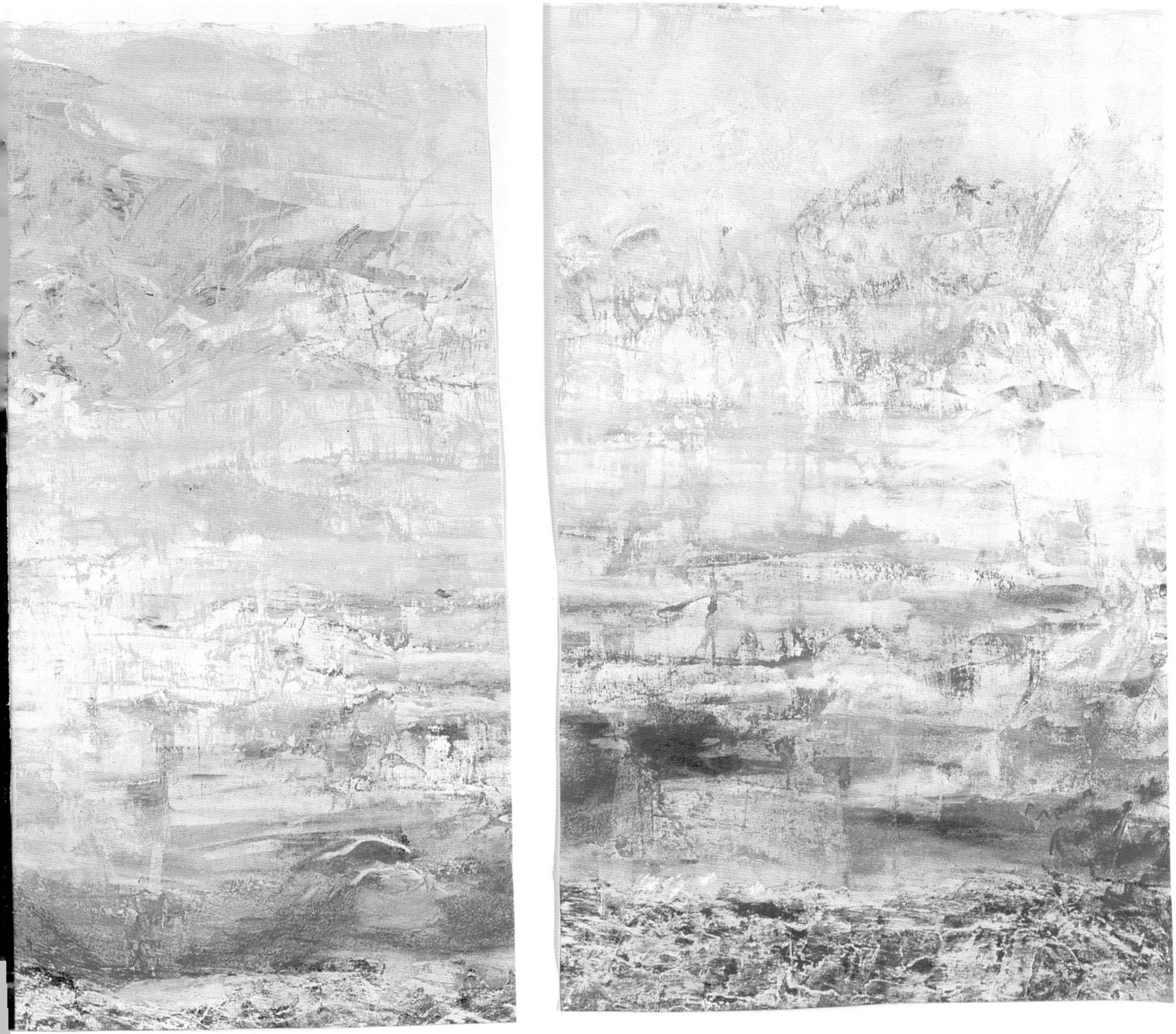

No one wrote a manual...

Breast cancer.

Mastectomy.

No estrogen.

Mein gott, this is hard. Harder than I expected. Time for psychotherapy, I finally admit to myself.

It is her voice on her answering machine. Thank God she is still in her office, still seeing clients. She who counseled with Stacy years ago during a custody battle. Her name is Leah. A psychologist for children, adolescents, families, and a woman reeling from breast cancer.

Mastectomy, again.

Breast cancer, again.

Renewed estrogen helps. Thank you, my doctors.

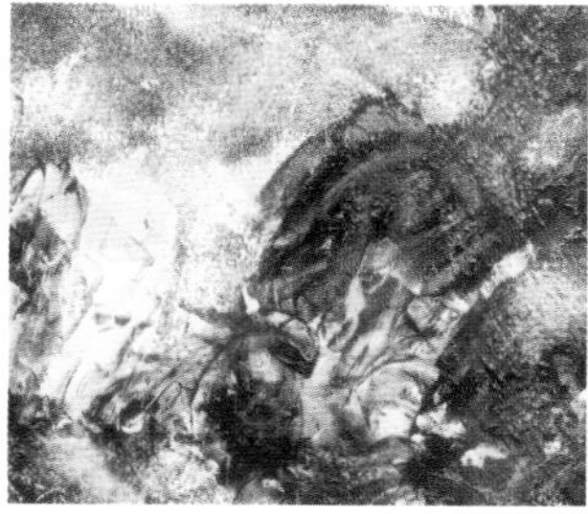

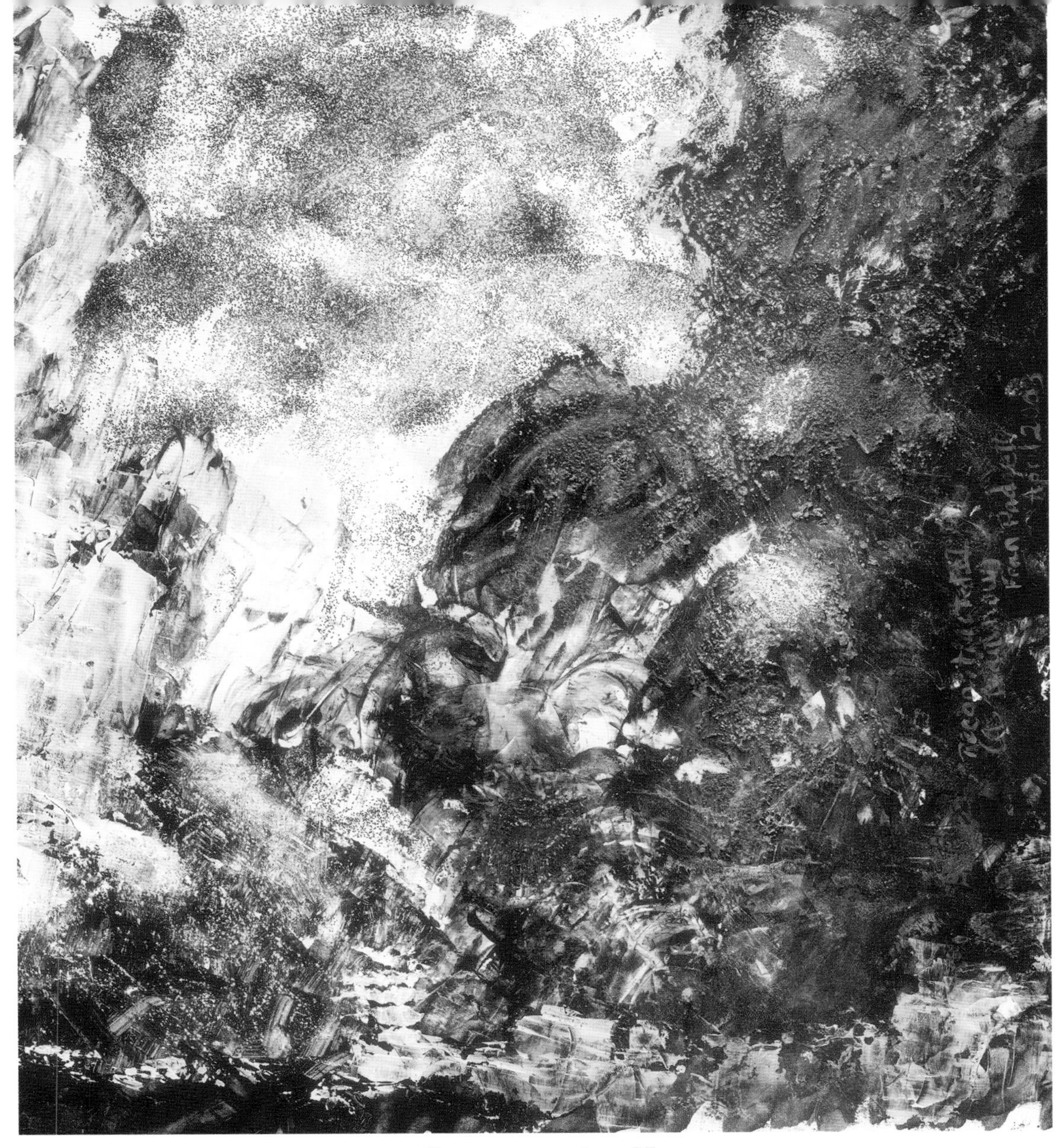

Reconstruction II

St. Guadaloupe

Pushing through the pain, god it gets hard some days.

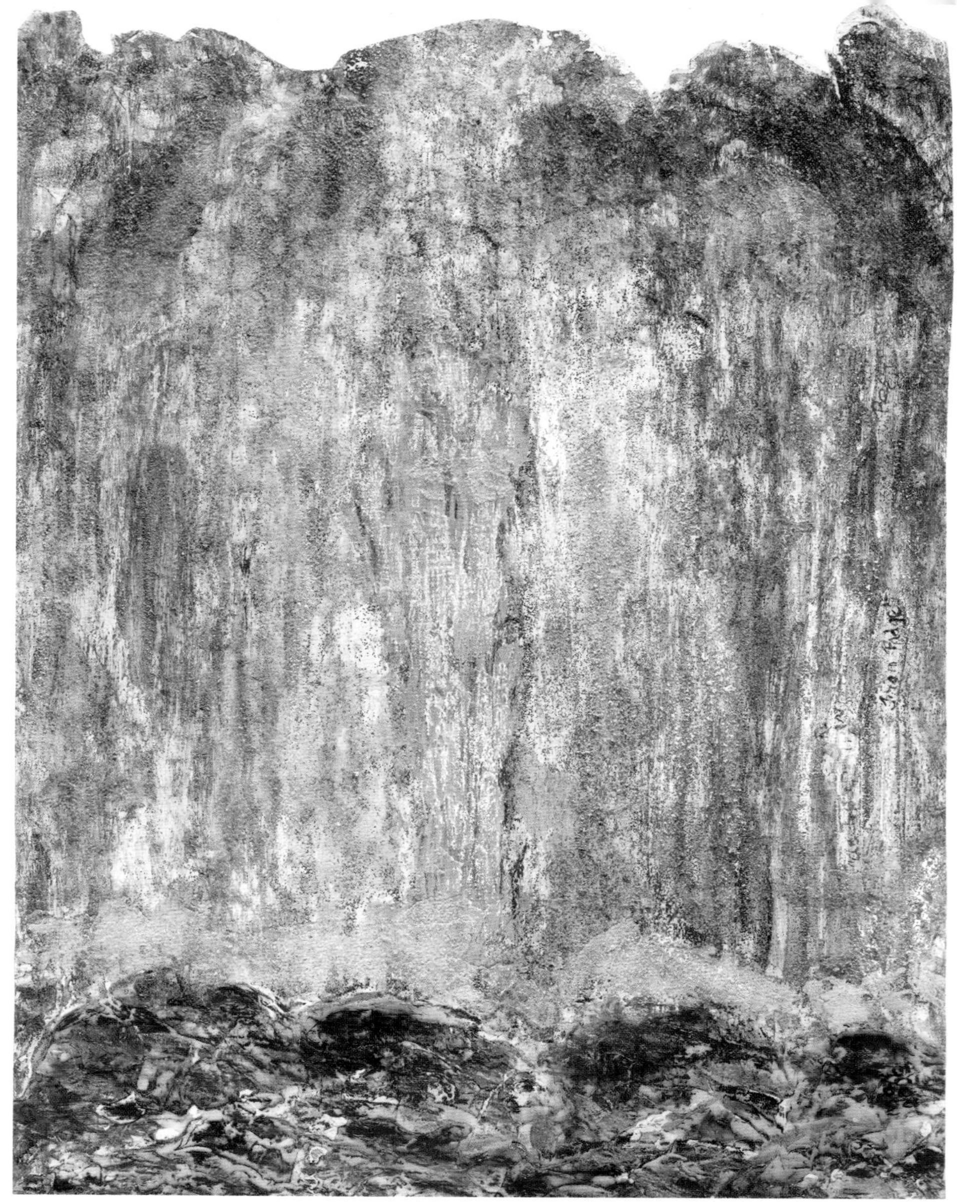

Reconstruction VIII
Waterfall
Fantasies, dreams, and visions, from where are they coming?

Leah's office becomes my oasis for sorting and sifting through a jangle of nerves and pain. Soothing my psyche, my soul, like water bathing a sorely stressed body.

Moving to live alone.

Leaving devastated a man who has always adored me.

"Leah, I don't know if I am doing this right. I only know my soul requires it. How do I tell him? What should I have said?"

"Fran, you are entering new territory. You are charting a new course for yourself. No one wrote a manual for you to go by."

Time moves on. I wonder if Leah might someday write that manual.

I can only hope.

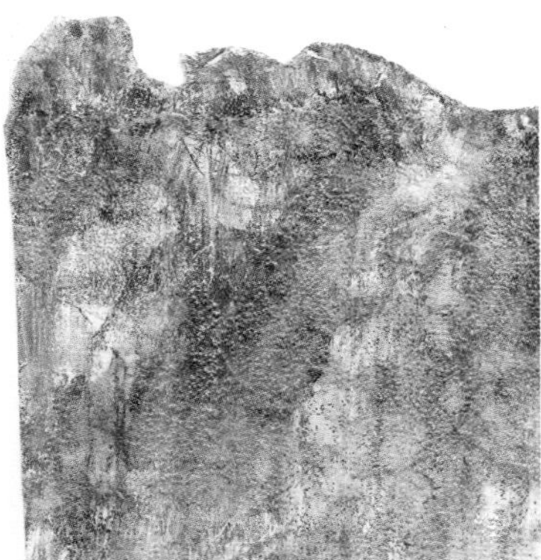

The next series

"Would you paint yourself as you are now?" I am asked.

"NO!" I replied.

But the question stayed in my head like a challenge. Putting my easel under the dining room skylight and filling the taboret with new pastels and acrylics, then choosing papers of random colors and sizes, I began exploring the subject of my different body.

Photographs taken in Montana gave me inspiration. Photographs taken at night at home gave me reference points. Gradually the paintings transitioned from exploratory to searching to a few "as I am now."

There are now 18 *Moving On* paintings. Unlike the *Sunrise* series that permanently concluded at 14, the *Moving On* series will be on-going for a while.

How many more? Only the soul of the artist knows and will say when to stop.

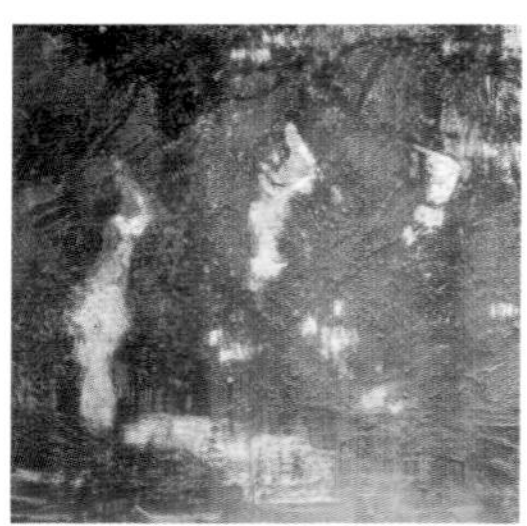

Reconstruction VI
X-Rays
I might as well stop looking for answers, there may not be any.

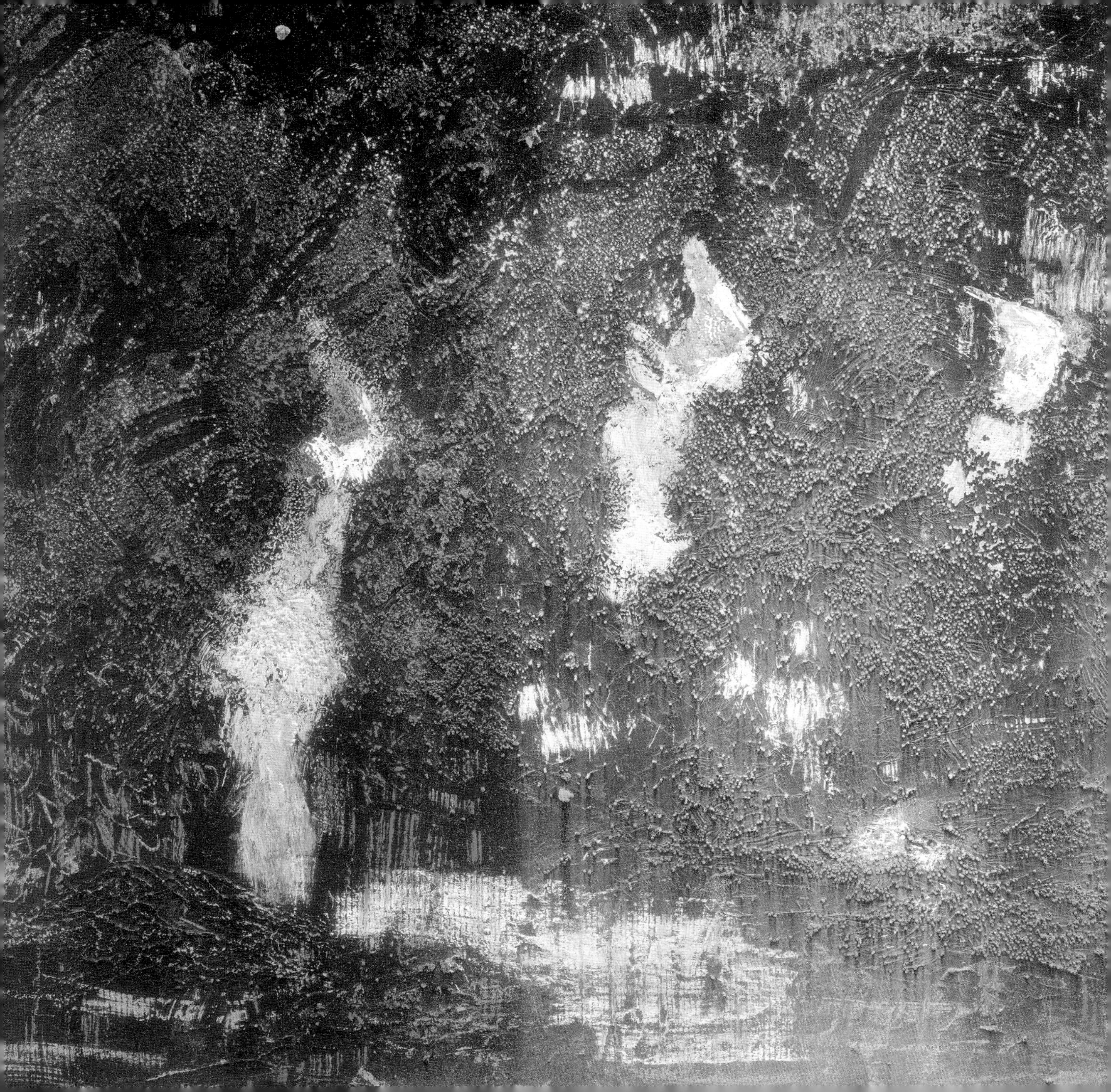

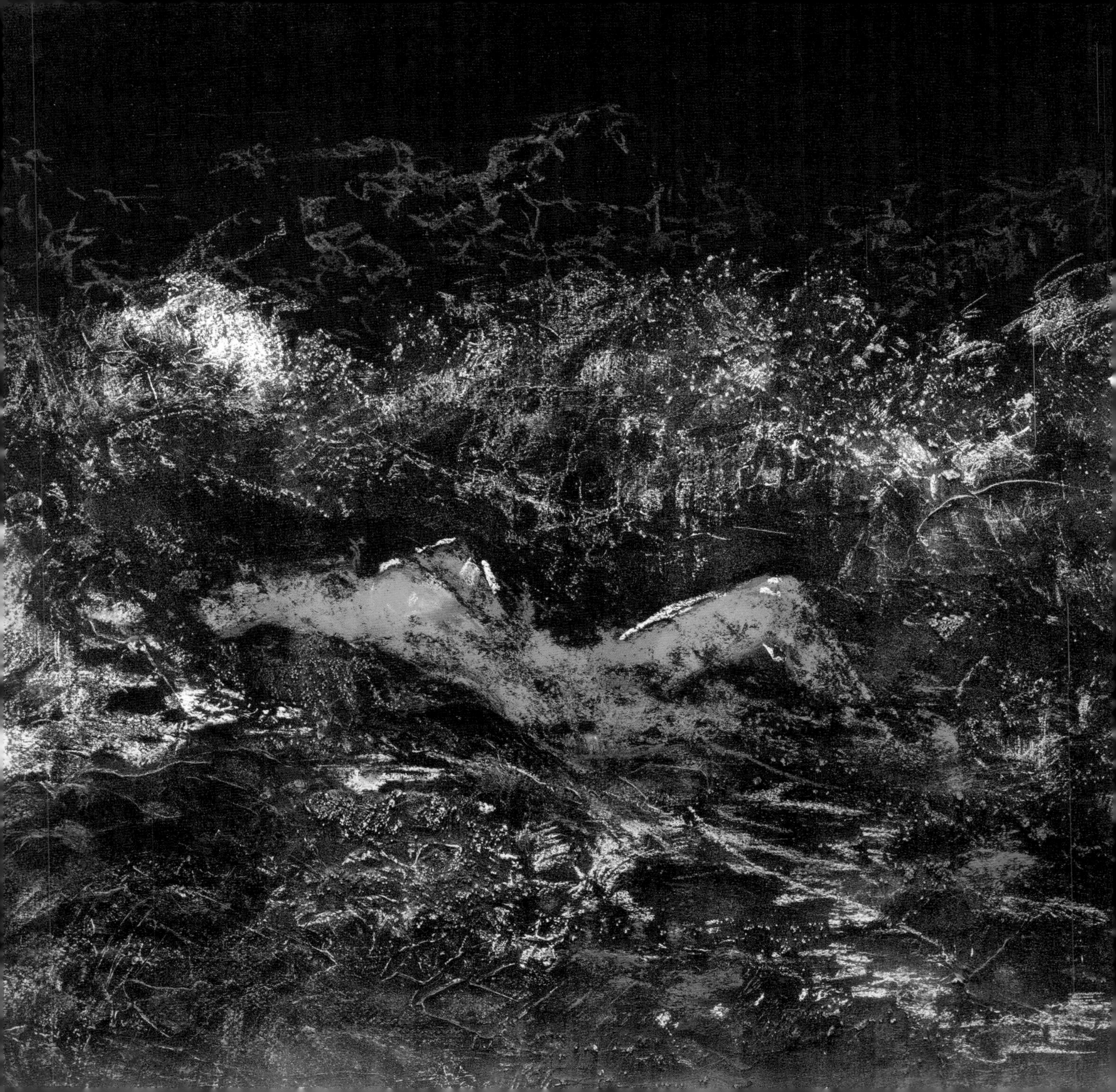

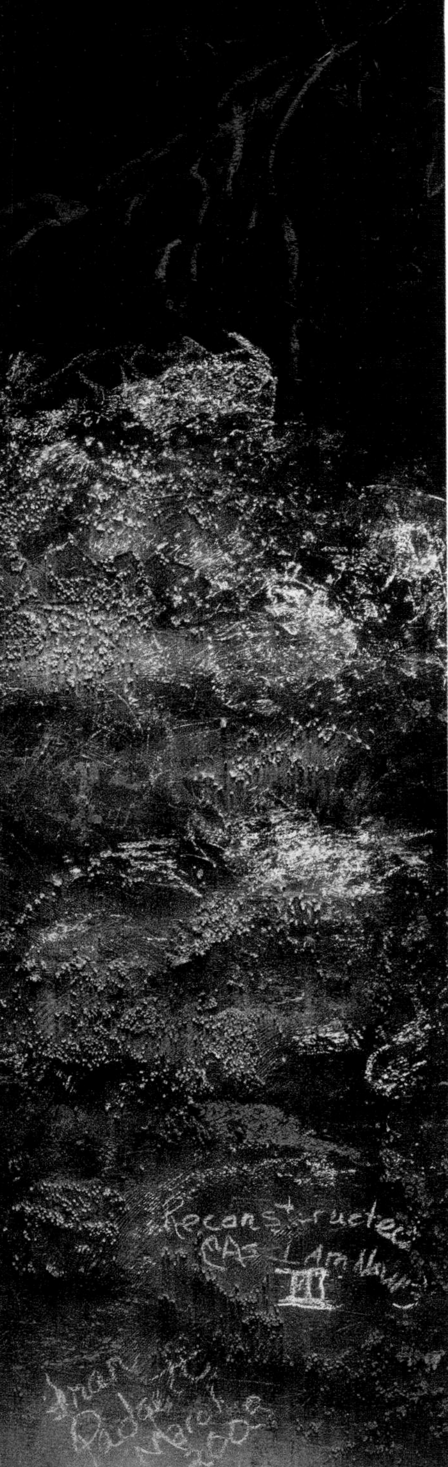

A reminder!

"Nancy," I said to my friend. "You won't believe what I have to do. Next week I am scheduled to meet with a tax review board to protest this outrageous increase in our property taxes. I have searched and struggled to get together as many supporting documents as I can find, write, print, or otherwise dream up. But I have no idea if it will all be enough to convince them that I'm right."

"Are the people on the board men or women?" Nancy asked.

"I've been told probably men."

"Well," Nancy said, "don't forget you now have CLEAVAGE!"

"Hey! That's right! I'll let you know how it goes!"

Reconstruction III
Rock Formation (black)
Silicone implants, so far the closest substitute for the real thing that man has invented (and I am thankful – they surely are better than two slash-y scars.)

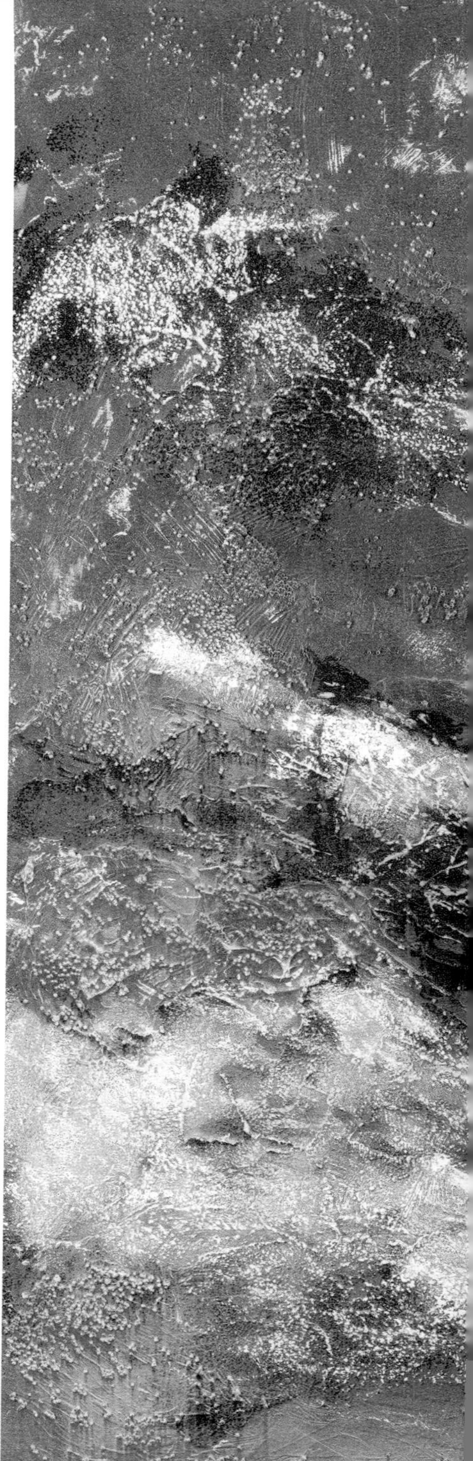

Reconstruction IV
Rock Formation (blue)
But I didn't expect to be quite so big!

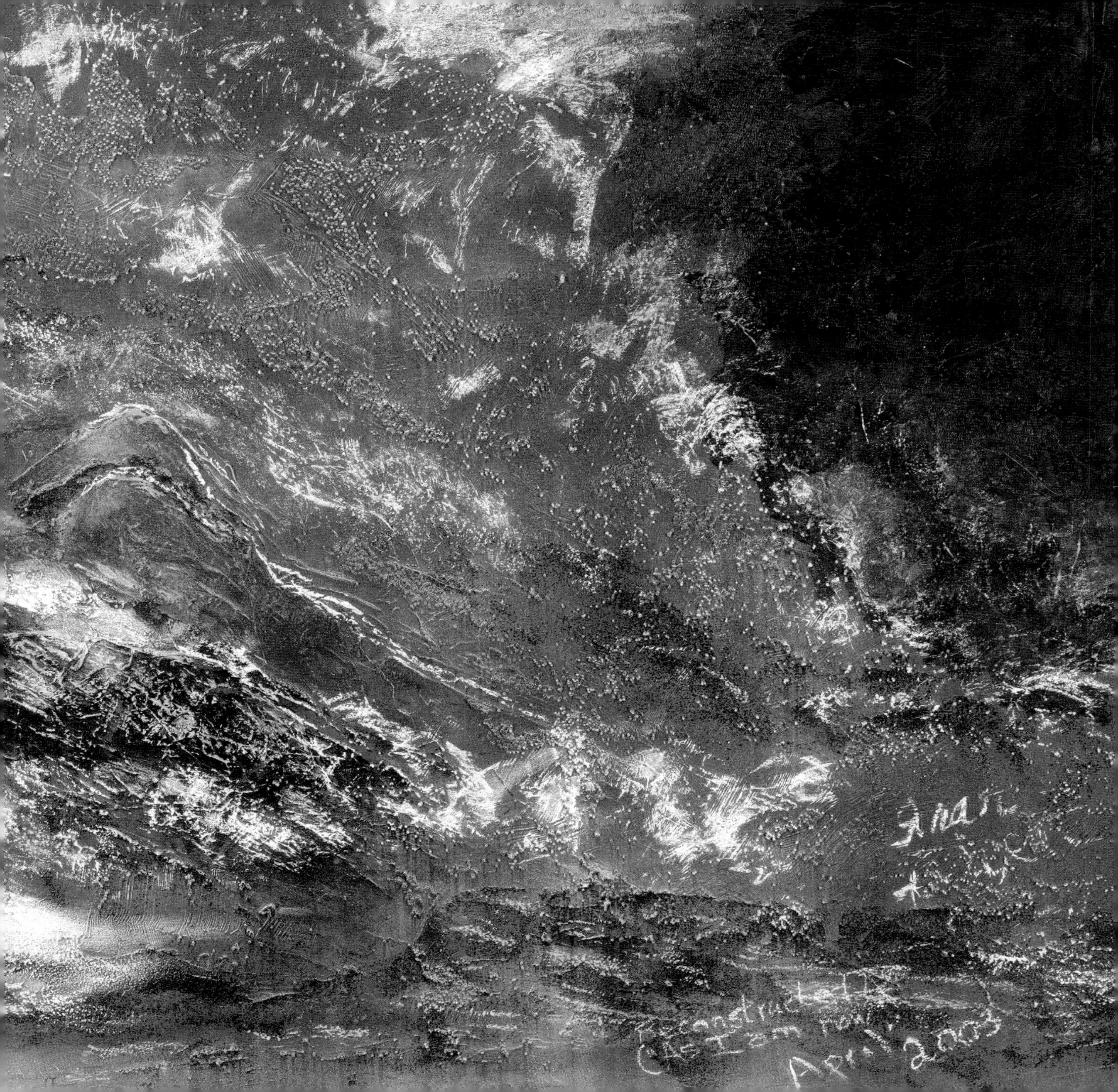

Are you the Genie?

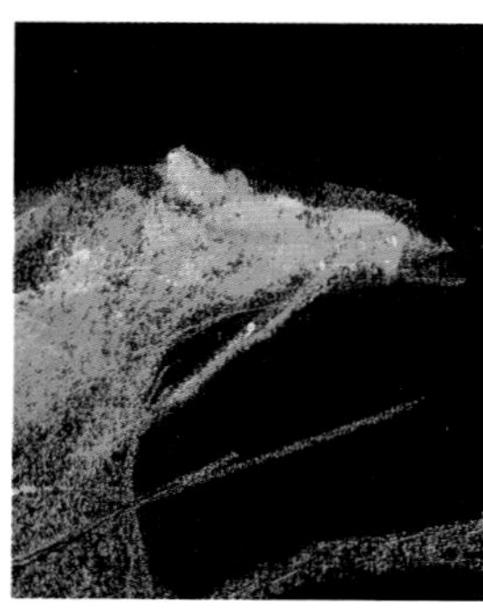

Strange but my Aladdin's Lamp looks like a weathervane…

He took the last swallow from his cocktail.

He pushed back from the table.

He rose from his chair.

He glowered and towered over me.

"Besides seeing me naked, what do you want from me?"

Through my mind flashed the children's book illustration of the Genie rising from Aladdin's lamp.

I leaned back in my chair a little, tilted my head back, cocked at an angle. *Yes,* I thought to myself. *There may be a little resemblance.*

"Are you the Genie? And do I get three wishes?" I smiled. He grinned ever-so-slightly.

"Okay. I want from you your friendship. I ask that you accept me as I am, meaning please accept my artistic quirkiness. I want to hear your soft and gentle laugh."

Later: "What you have asked of me is NOTHING."

I know, my friend. I know it may seem like nothing to you. They mean the world to me right now.

Years later: What I asked of you seemed nothing at the time, but one by one you took away my wishes. Do you realize, though, that you have left me with an Aladdin's Lamp? It is your cherished weathervane remnant of a trotting horse with sulky.

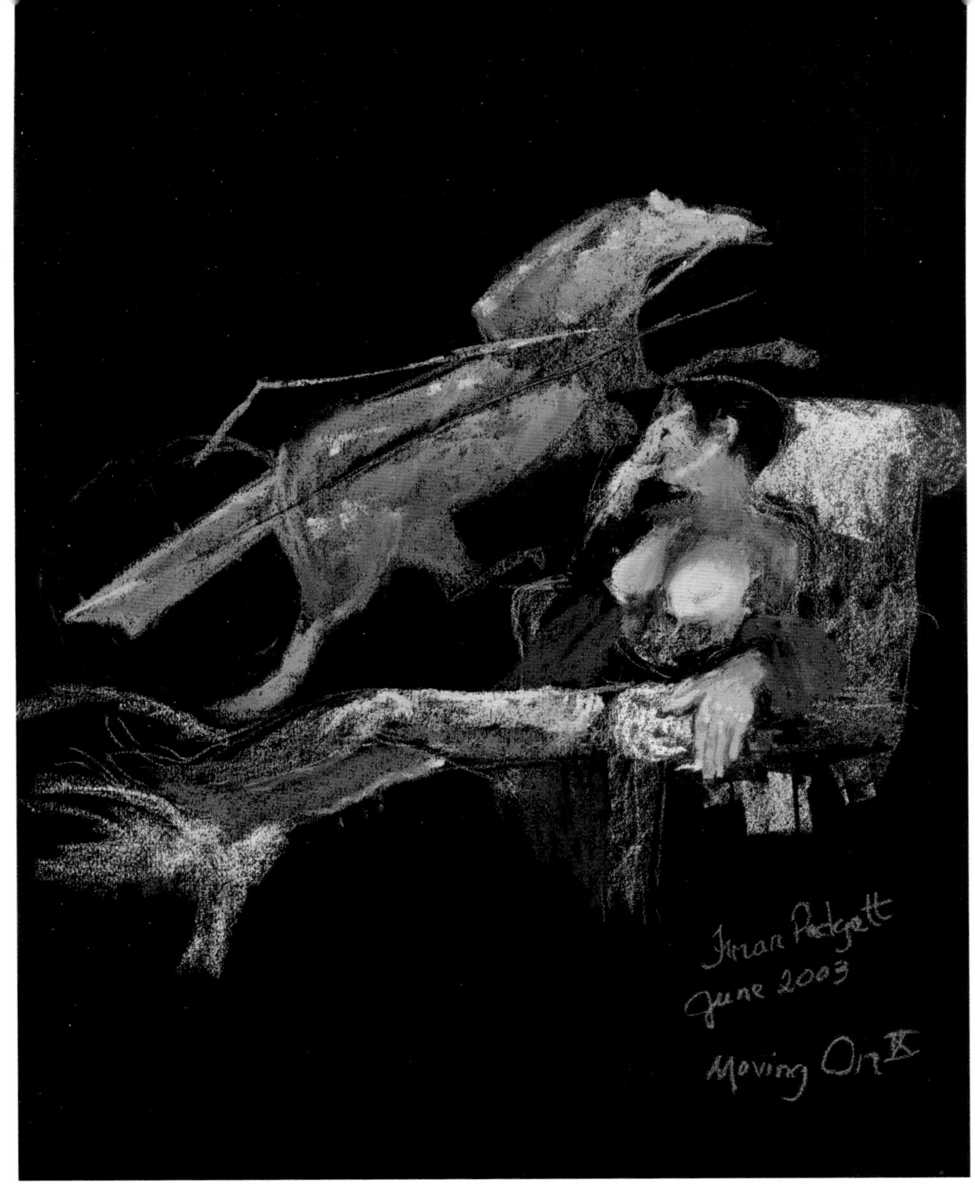

Reconstruction X

("As I am Now")

The Weathervane

New paths, new directions, will the wind be at my back?

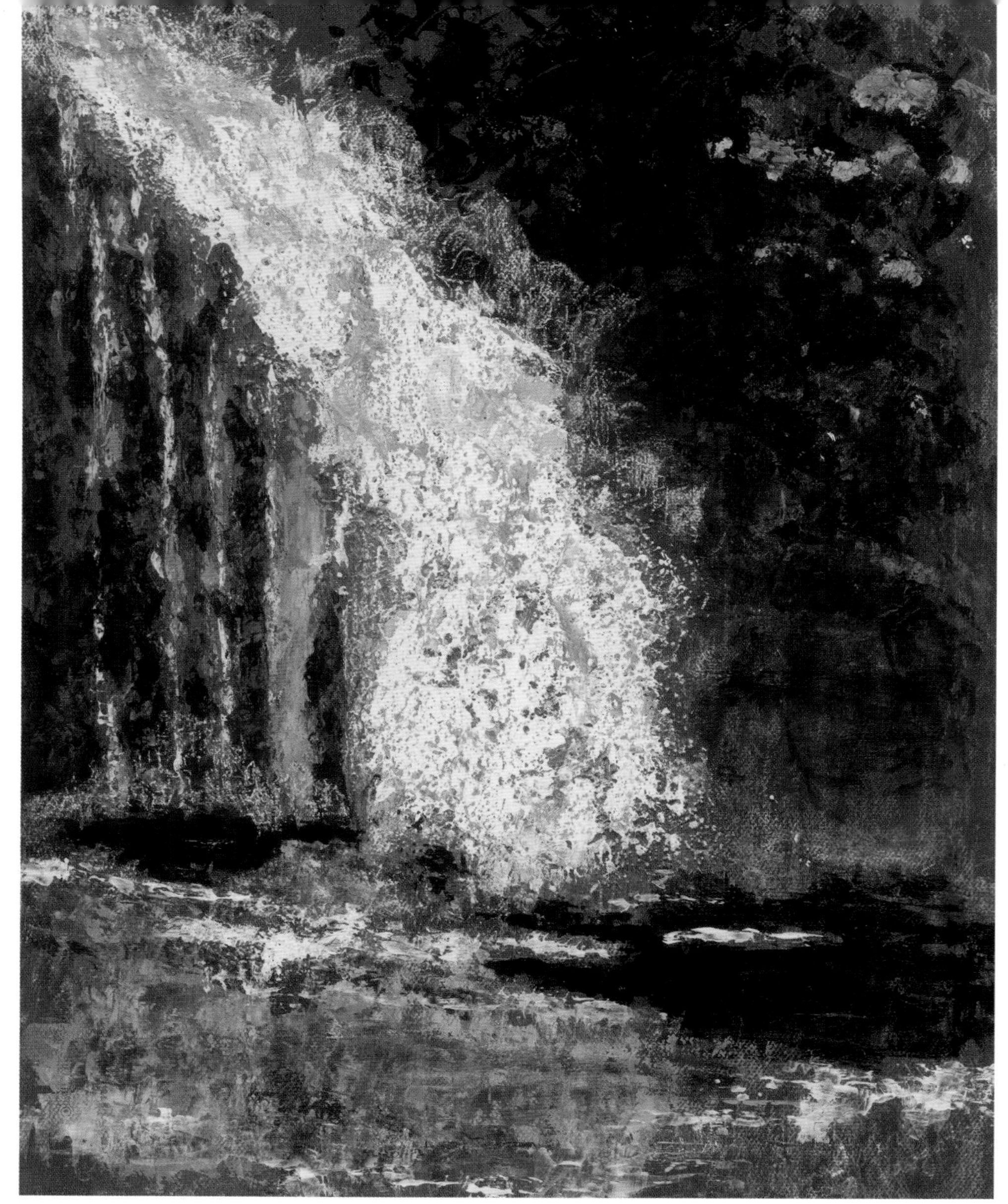

Reconstruction IX

Woodsy Waterfall

And what do you mean?

A blessing or a curse?

My new special friend said, "I described you to someone and that person thought I should ask you. 'What do you want from me?'"

He seemed genuinely perplexed. Maybe no one ever wanted to be "just a friend." Maybe his other acquaintances only wanted favors and "freebies" from his company.

I hesitated. *[Well, here goes nothing, I thought.]*

"I have a nearly photographic memory. Sometimes it feels like a blessing, sometimes more like a curse." I paused. "But could I see you undressed and memorize your body?"

My new special friend blushed. And was uncharacteristically speechless. I guess no one had ever asked for a favor or "freebie" like that.

After a long pause he regained his voice, "For a painting?"

I smiled to myself. "Oh, maybe. Someday."

The "Lady" in black – a new companion

"Dede," my granddaughter Stacy said to me, over and over, "I have to have my own dog. Please, Dede, please."

Her words sent us on a "mission" to find just the right dog. Not too big, not too small. Not too young, not too old. Not too nervous, not too shaggy. And healthy. And housebroken. The mission took us to a "no-kill shelter" that "gives dogs away" for a small donation of $100.00.

And at the no-kill shelter was a beautiful black dog who eagerly jumped into the truck and onto Stacy's lap.

The shelter people were happy to get the donation. They tried to tell us Lady was a black Lab. Actually, she is obviously purebred English Setter, in the rare all black.

Stacy's psychiatrist told Stacy to "take care of the little doggie that is inside you."

And now Dede takes care of the derelict dog.

Reconstruction XIII

Lost and Found

It gives me peace to know that you put my memory in the safe place that only you know where to find me.

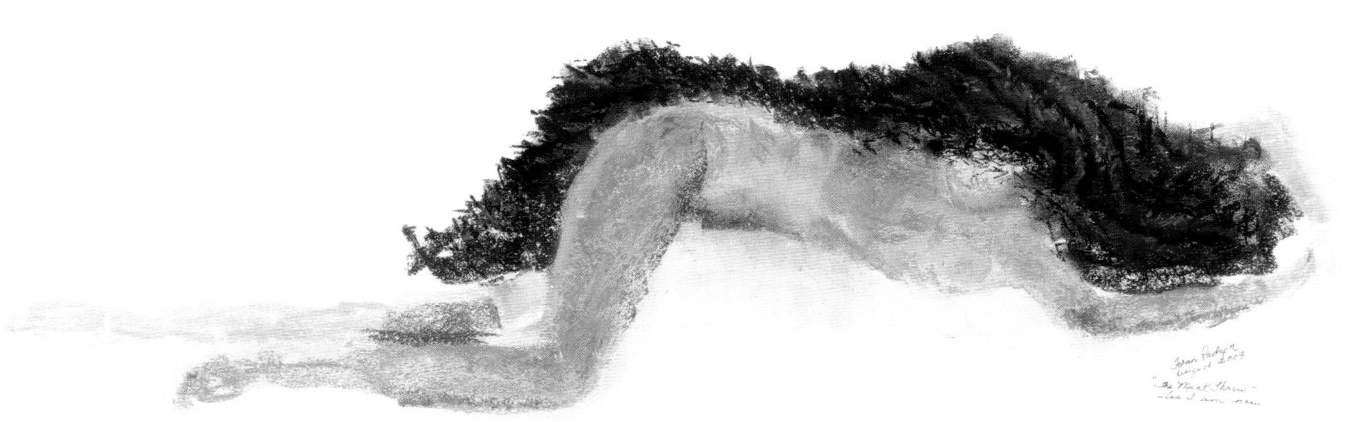

Fran's revenge...

What is it like to drive a "**HOT**" **red truck**? A customized GMC Sierra lengthened, lowered, leathered and chromed? Big tires, special wheels and chrome tail pipes, hitches front and rear. I've looked and looked and can't find another one like it in the city of Houston.

"Don't you like your Jaguar any more?" A very fine sedan in British racing green from my husband, given to me the year before breast cancer.

Since living in Houston I have driven matronly, sedate sedans, while Texas cowboys in their fancy pickups with bad driving manners zip and zoom around me driving infuriatingly fast.

Now I drive a **HOT RED TRUCK**, the envy of males (and some females). And now Texas cowboys don't zoom around me. They slow down and admire.

This truck is Fran's revenge!

Reconstruction XII
("As I am Now")
The Mink Throw
Needing comfort, needing luxury.

"Spreading the word"

What marvelous pages come from the pen of the P.R. lady! She takes words and sentences from my conversations with her and repeats them, only better.

She calls herself Czarina. I call her my Colonel Parker.

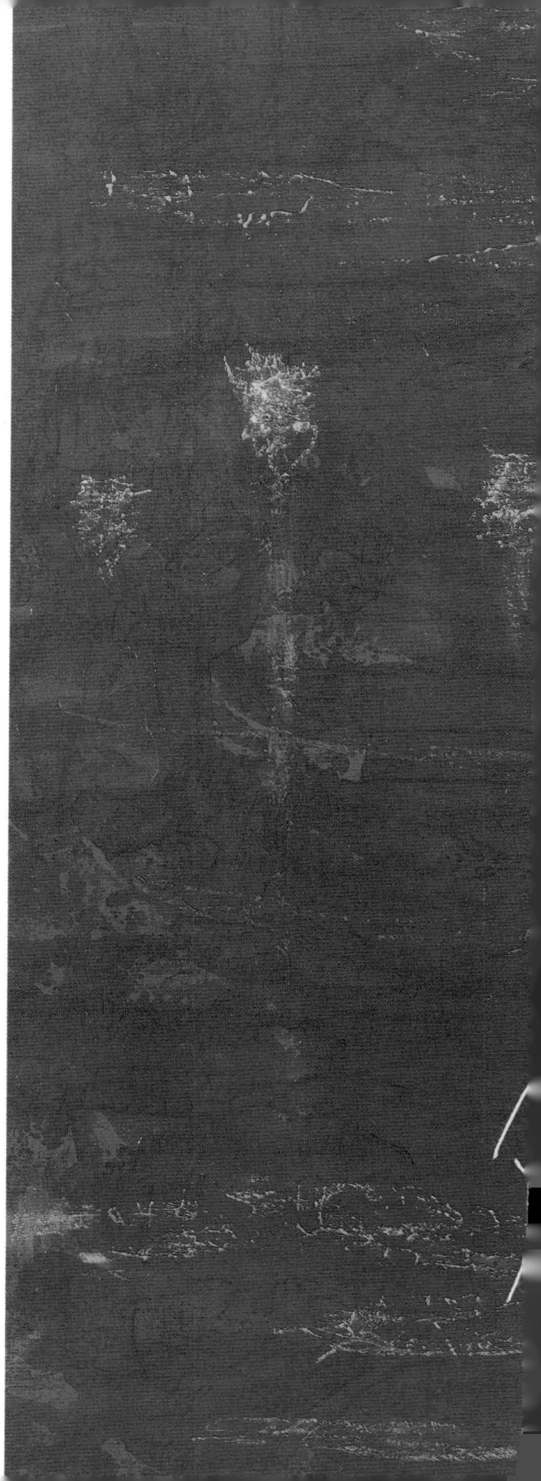

Reconstruction XVII
The Bridge from There to Here
Follow your heart, pursue your dreams, and
the bridge will appear, you see.

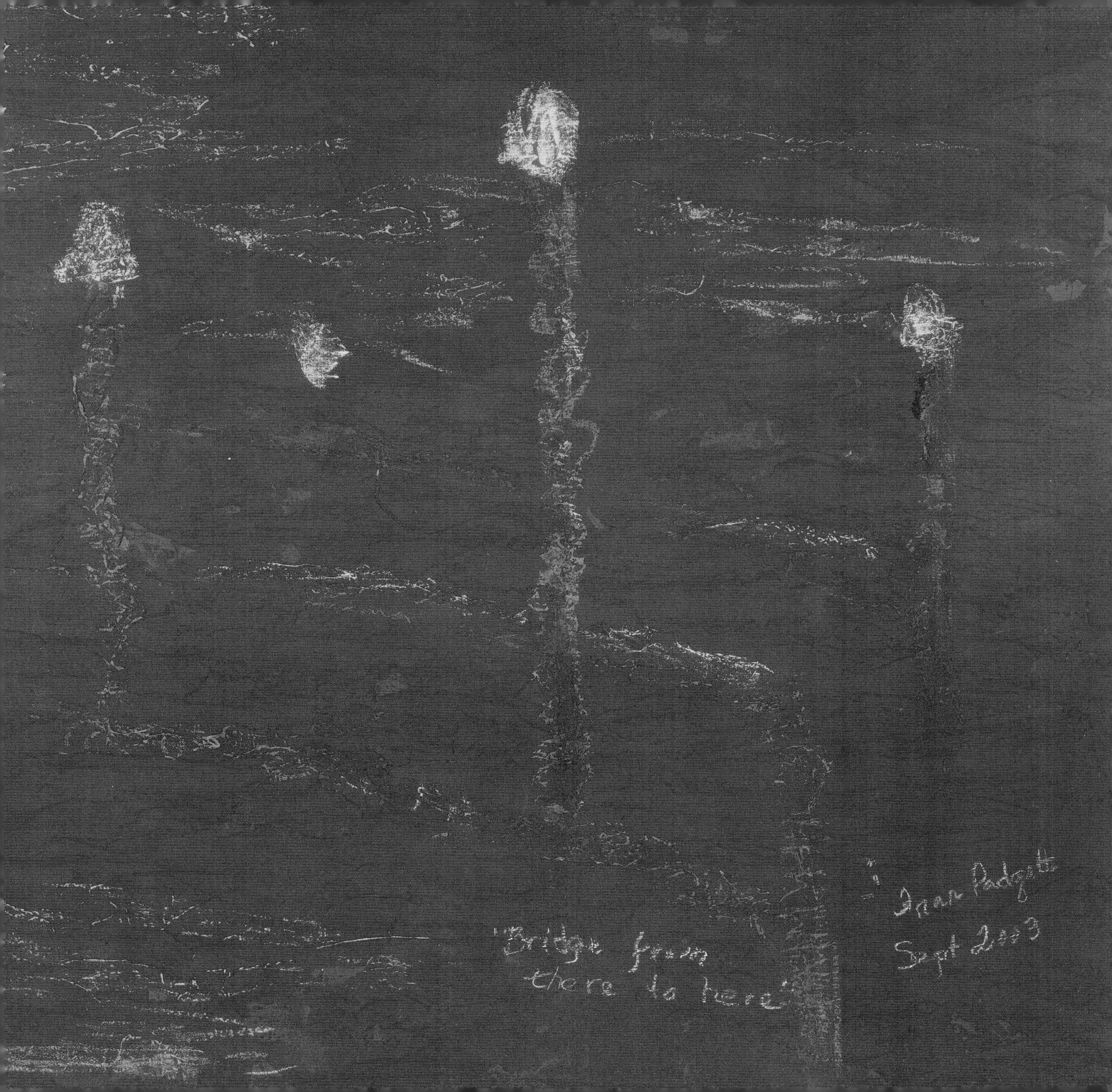
"Bridge from
there to here"
Sept 2003

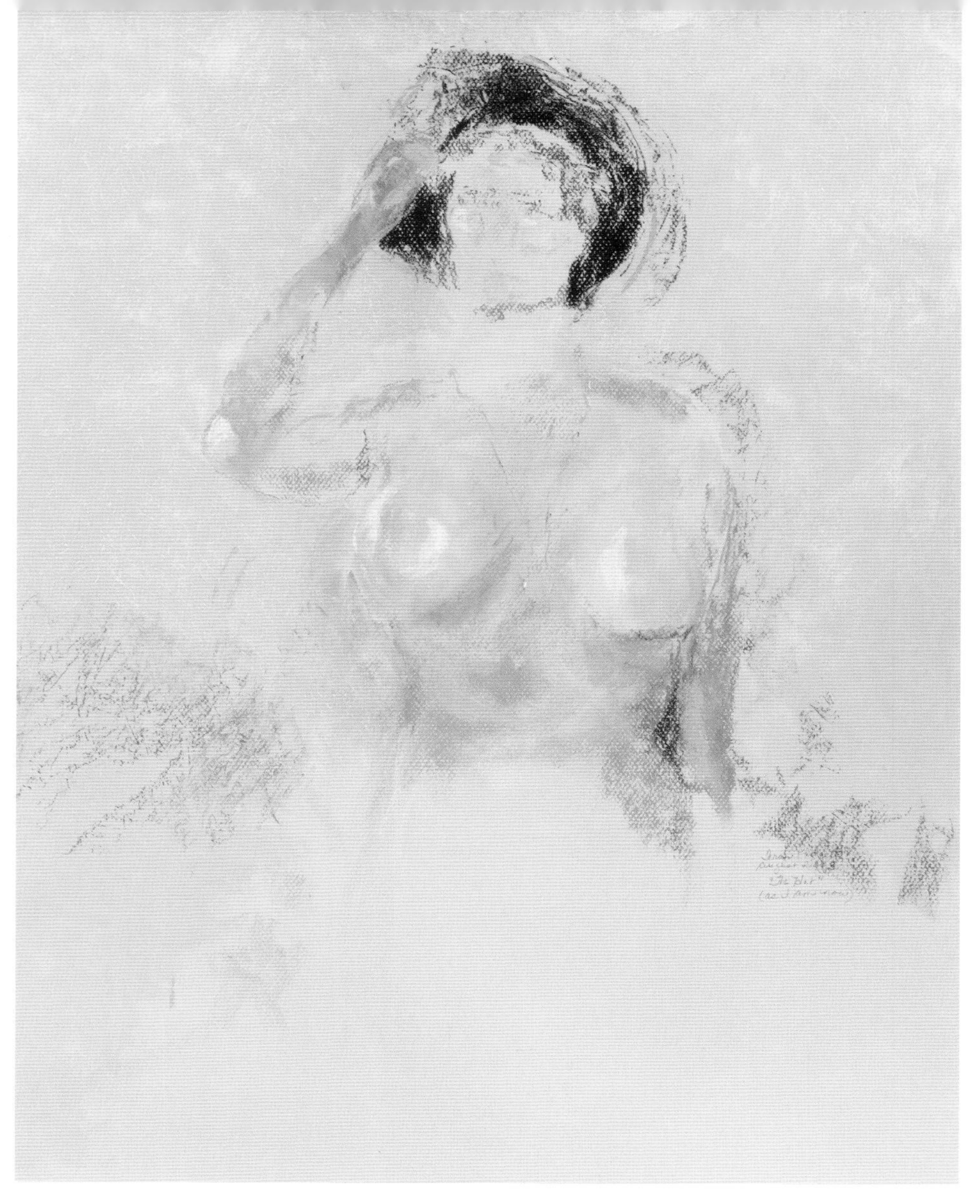

Reconstruction XIV
("As I am Now")
The Hat
A new hat…new reason to go shopping!

Trading a gold band for a gold chain necklace

June 2002

"See this hand?" My husband gently held my left hand out, palm side down, to show his best friend — the friend who had been the best man at our wedding and had handed the ring to the groom to put on the bride's ring finger.

"She took her wedding band off. She hasn't worn it in months."

December 2002

Opening the small Christmas gift box, I find a new gold chain with a diamond heart. The card is signed, "I love you."

"I love you, too," I told him.

I have worn it ever since.

One week later I moved to my new house.

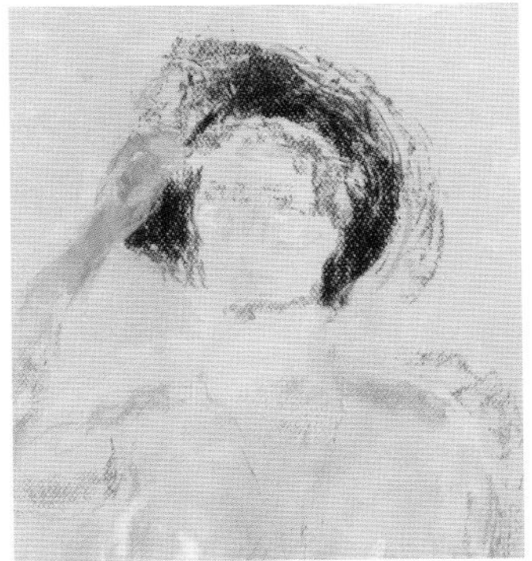

Head over heels over Felix...

Stacy and I love horses. I'm told this love is in our genes because my great-grandfather raised thoroughbreds and Morgans.

Stacy rides with strength and skill — a hunter-jumper equestrienne. Her first horse was Beckon To Me, an affectionate and lively bay mare, whose stable name was "Becky." Her second horse was Snap To It, a tall, chestnut thoroughbred gelding with spirit and an attitude, whose stable name was "Snapple."

My therapist had encouraged me to spend time pursuing passionate loves. So I would go to the stable where Snapple and Stacy fly ever so high over jumps, trotting and cantering in precise patterns around the arena.

It has been years and years, but I yearn to see if I can ride again. Stacy's trainer, Julie, agrees to let me try riding on Felix. Felix is a school horse, dependable, gentle, even-tempered. And so old his stable name is "Grampa."

Julie lends me a comfortable saddle. Nacho, a stable hand, helps me with the tacking up. Carolyn, a substitute teacher, patiently assists me to ride Felix around the arena in gentle walks and a few short trots.

"KEEP HEELS DOWN," I am instructed. It is of paramount importance that I stay *mounted*. I must not fall. No sprains, no broken bones. Mastectomies and reconstruction require all the doctor and hospital visits this woman wants to deal with!

After a few riding lessons, Carolyn and I relax. And so does my Grampa Felix by putting his head down. And there I go in a slow-motion summersault over his head, landing flat on my back, THUD, in the soft dirt track. Carolyn is shocked and distressed, but only my pride and composure are hurt. Emergency room definitely not needed.

As soon as I get home, I tell Stacy about my slow motion, head-over-heels tumble from Grampa Felix.

"Dede, I have told you and told you, KEEP YOUR HEELS DOWN!

"I am making you a sign to wear on your back when you ride!"

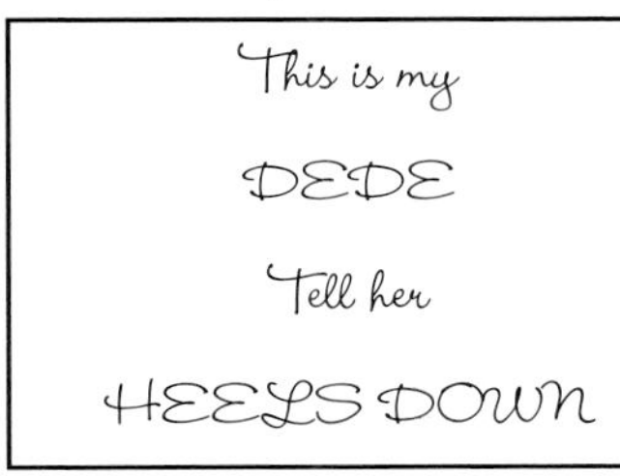

Reconstruction XV

The Fox and The Bear; Guardian Spirits in the Air

Unbidden images…why do they keep coming and what do they mean?

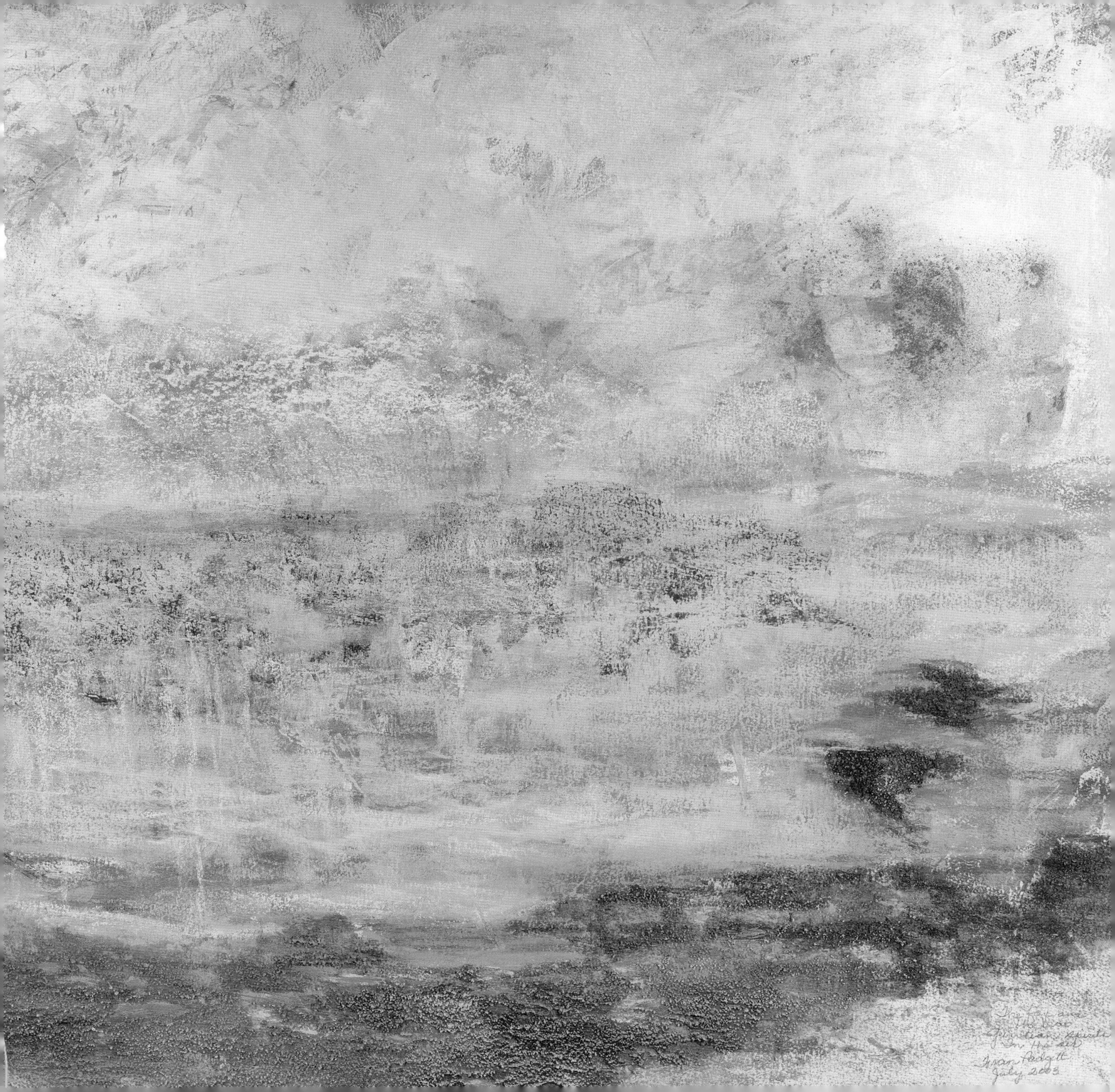
July 2003

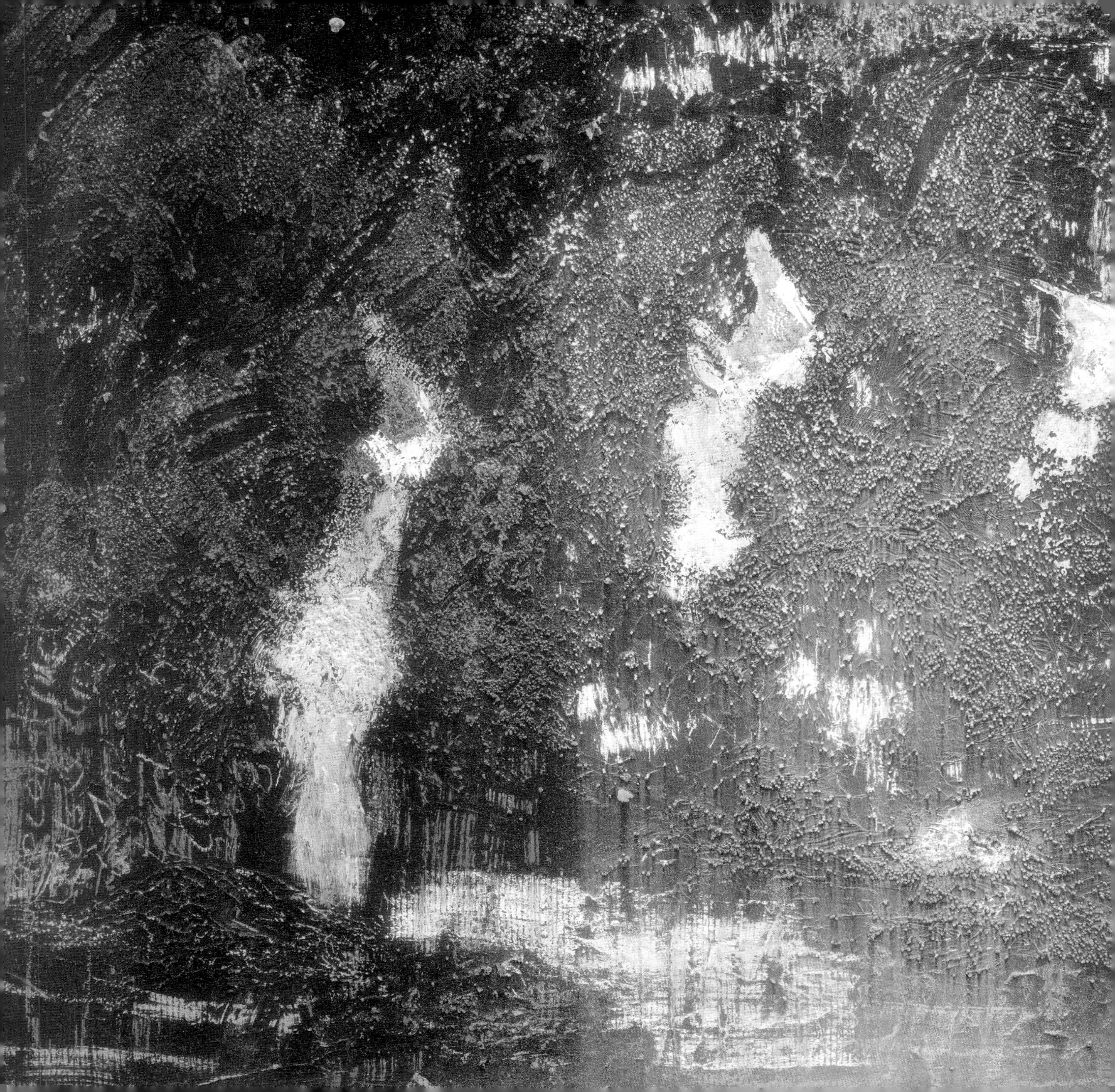

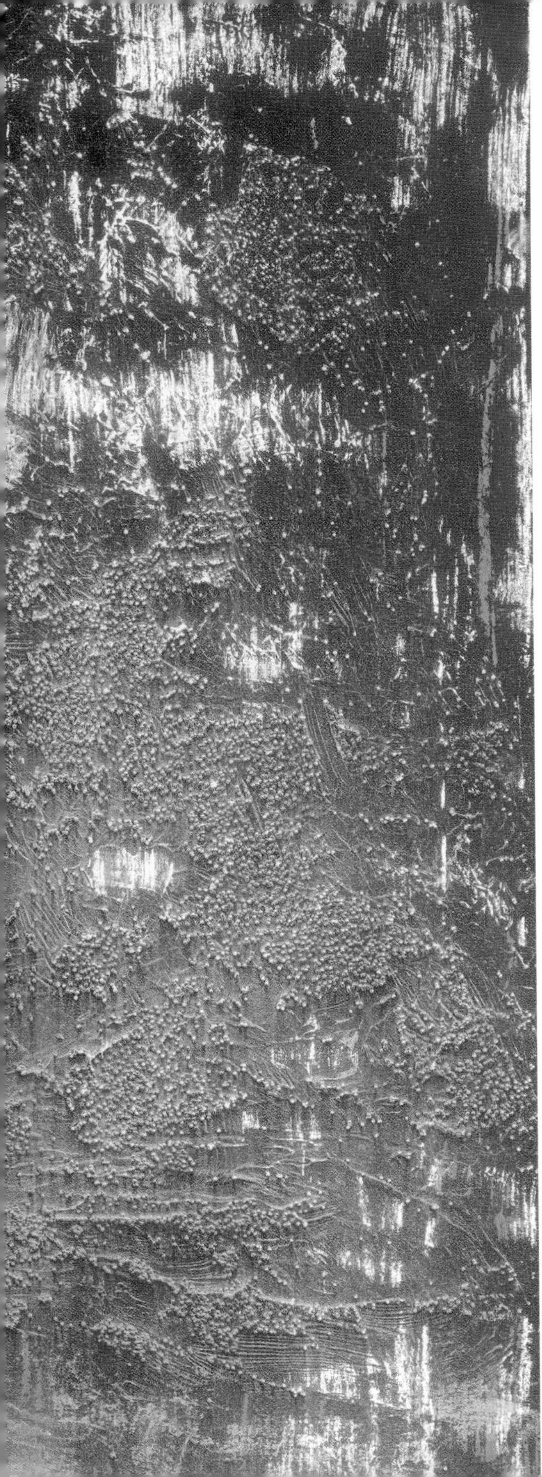

"Be able to be alone..."

On the label of the Tchaikovsky CD, the first music played the first night at my new house...

> *"Be able to be alone.*
> *Lose not the advantage of solitude,*
> *and the society of thyself."*
> *— Sir Thomas Browne*

I don't know much about you, Sir Thomas. In fact I have never heard of you before. Someday I'll look for your biography. I'd like to know more about someone who wrote the very words I had been thinking.

Reconstruction V
X-Rays (with subliminal face)
Fantasies and visions, what is the reality?

The word is out!!!

"The new neighbor is an ARTIST!"

The looks on their faces let me read their minds. "Eccentric…Quirky… Weird…Different."

I now reside in a small enclave of 39 townhomes. Word has spread fast, it seems. The new neighbor paints nudes!!! And probably even paints while nude. You never know!

The doorbell rings. With Stacy standing behind me, I open the door to a middle-aged, slightly paunchy, dark haired man, who is holding out an envelope.

"This is yours. It was in my mailbox. I thought I would bring it to your door instead of returning it to the post office. I live just two doors away."

His head is trying to see around me and Stacy, into our studio, his neck stretching out like a long swivel, his eyes big and roaming, all without taking any forward step.

"That's really nice of you. Thanks so much. I expect we'll be seeing you around the neighborhood." My words are hopefully polite enough to slowly close the door.

"Stacy, did it seem to you that he was trying to be nosey?"

"Oh, yes! He looked at you and saw big boobs. He looked at me and saw big boobs. He wanted to see more."

We double over in gales of laughter. Some faces even adolescents can read. And some adolescents can read faces better than weird artists can.

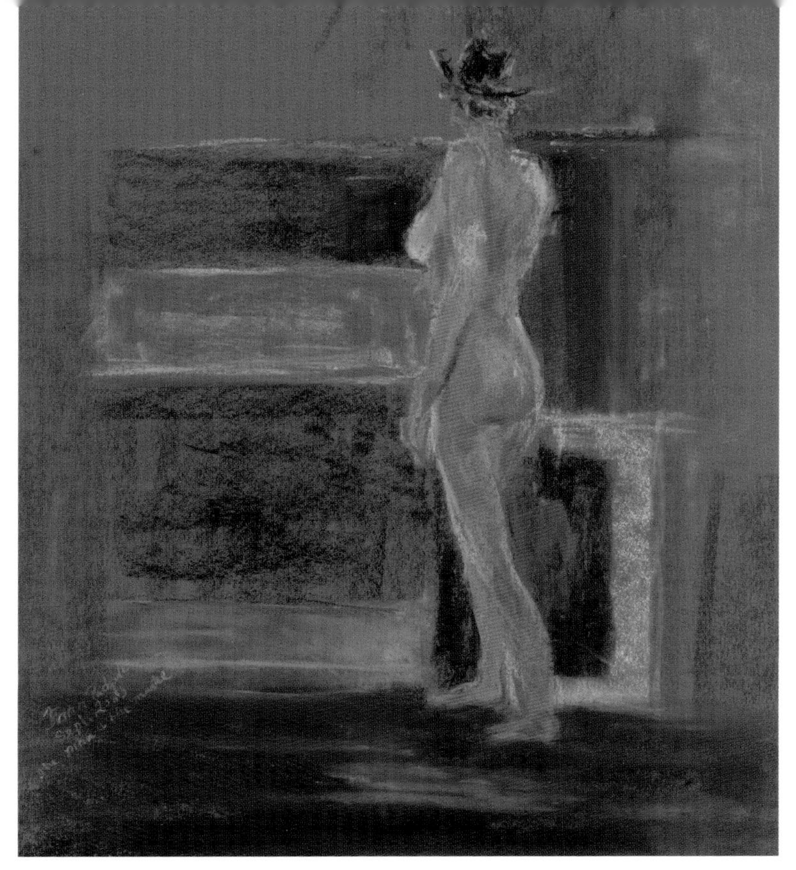

Reconstruction XVIII
("As I am Now")
The Man and the Mantel
Not showing my face yet.

Words that strengthen,
praise that sustains...

My friends have come to the gallery exhibit of *Sunrise to Sunrise*. These nude self-portraits, these paintings of pain, are a farewell to my body as it was before mastectomies.

I see their tears.

I try to not show that I am quivering. I turn to the wall and pretend to take a sip of wine.

I feel more than see his presence at my back. His arm goes gently across my shoulders.

In the softest, kindest voice, he said, “I am proud of you.”

Oh, my friend. No one has ever in my life said that to me.

My body stiffens with the strength of those words. I turn back around to my friends. I smile at them and hug them.

I thank my friends for coming and wish them good evening as they leave. Everyone is gone, the gallery empty. I go home and find his note of praise and encouragement. He wrote:

> *'One day I hope the words come to me to describe to you what this weekend means to me. I've known you possess many gifts and blessings but to witness so many of them in one afternoon was overwhelming. Your courage, love, understanding and selflessness are an inspiration to me. Thank you.'*

Oh, my friend, my friend. Those special words still see me through many long hours of doubt and uncertainty. I thank you.

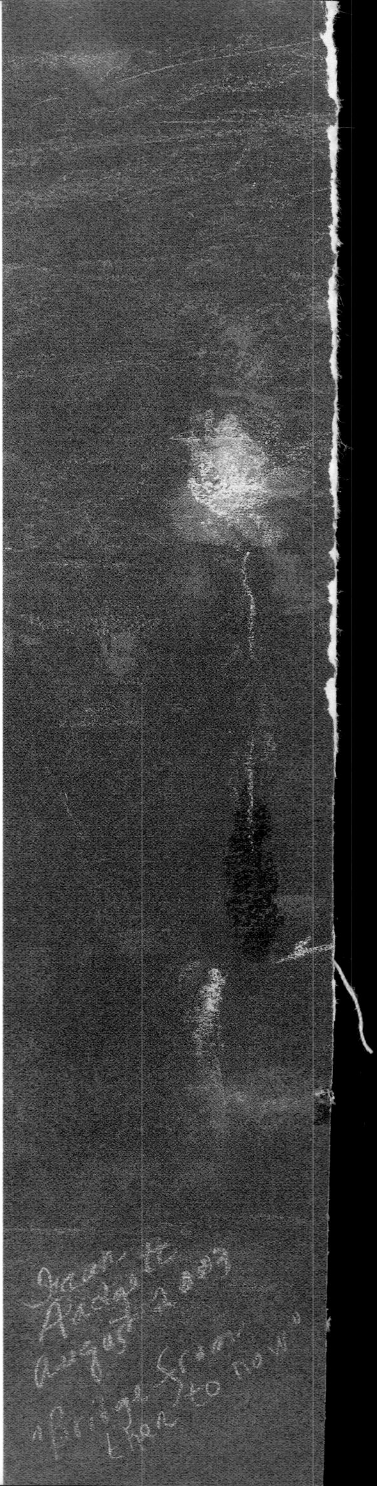

Reconstruction XVI

The Bridge From Then to Now

My special friend: You were my bridge from then to now;
You held my hand, you lighted my way

I will never forget.

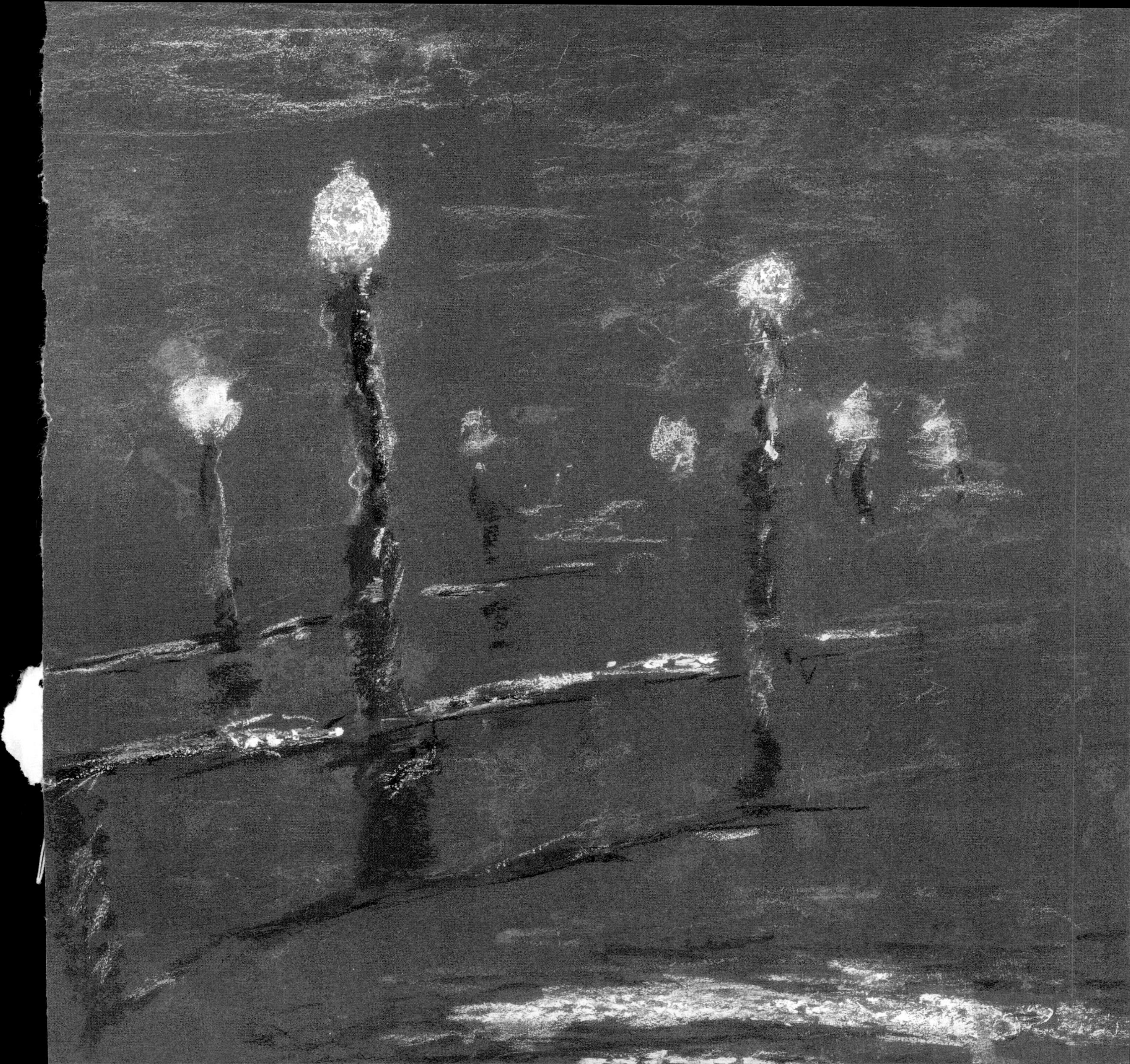

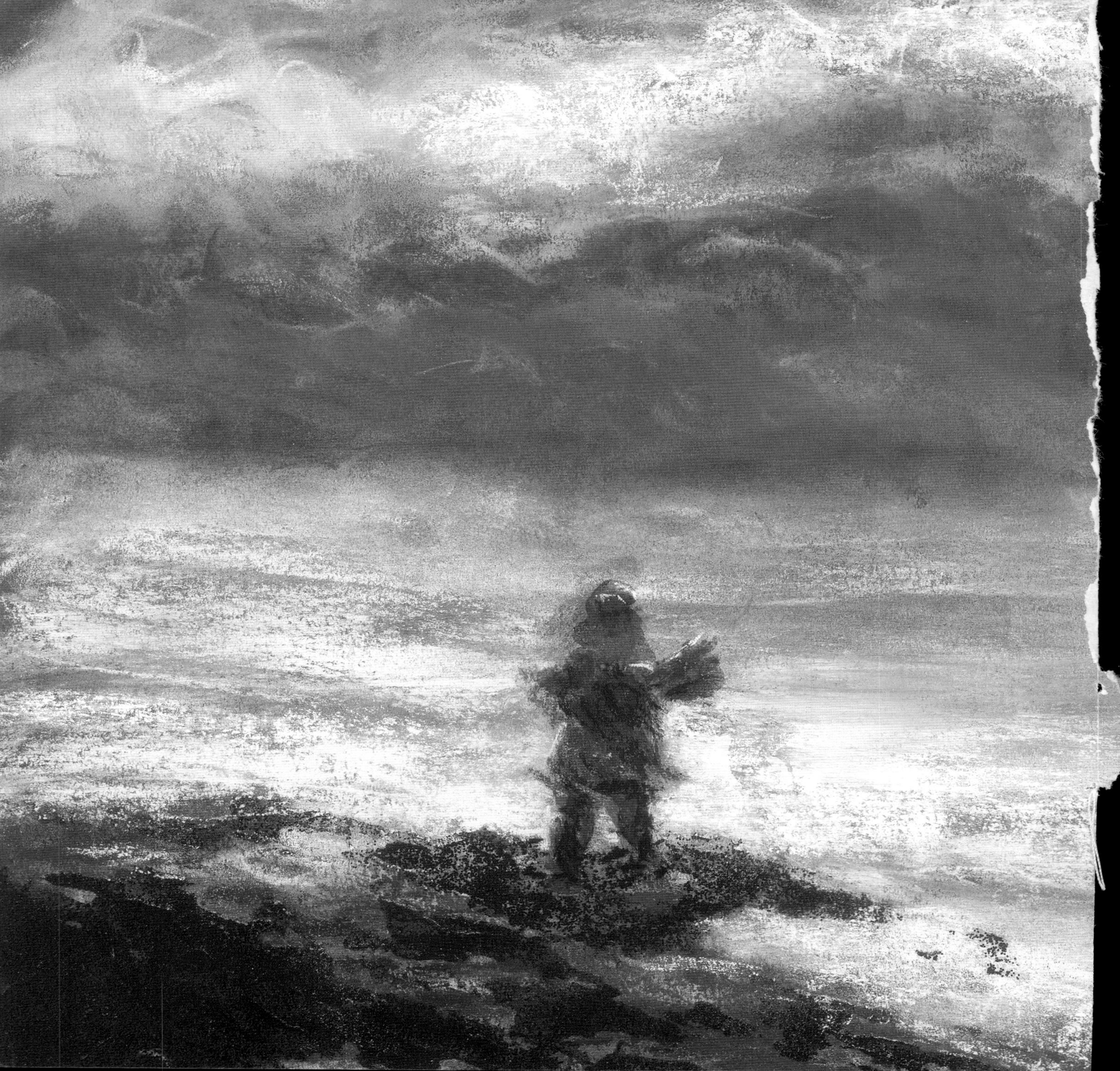

Reconstruction XI
The Wave
Wondering how far away to go.

EPILOGUE

"Please read it one more time," he requested, "as though it has been a long, long time since you've seen it."

Slowly, methodically I re-read these pages, as my publisher had asked. I saw that his discerning eye and gentle hands had rearranged the pain and emotions therein into a gift I can offer with humility and hope to share with you — the impact of breast cancer on one woman taking a road in life less traveled.

GUIDE TO PAINTINGS

PAGE	TITLE	SUB-TITLE	SIZE	MEDIA
4	Sunrise I		12" h x 19" w	Pastel on pastel paper
37	Sunrise II		22" h x 30" w	Pastel on watercolor paper
7	Recovery I	Caught Unaware	20" h x 13" w	Pastel on pastel paper
8	Recovery II	Dammit	21" h x 21" w	Pastel on pastel paper
10	Recovery III	My Camellias (Bloom in December)	12" h x 13" w	Pastel on pastel paper
12	Recovery IV	The Silver Chains	18" h x 12" w	Pastel on pastel paper
14	Recovery V	The Dark Window	17" h x 23" w	Pastel on pastel paper
16	Recovery VI	Facing the Garden Fence	25" h x 19" w	Pastel on pastel paper
21	Recovery VII	Bright Sun but No Warmth	25" h x 19" w	Pastel on pastel paper
23	Recovery VIII	Don't Touch Me!	19" h x 25" w	Pastel on pastel paper
25	Recovery IX	The Old Ficus Tree	25" h x 19" w	Pastel on pastel paper
27	Recovery X	The Tallow Tree	25" h x 19" w	Pastel on pastel paper
31	Recovery XI	The Gold Charm	21" h x 16" w	Pastel on pastel paper
34	Recovery XII	Seated	19" h x 22" w	Pastel on pastel paper

PAGE	TITLE	SUB-TITLE	SIZE	MEDIA
43	Reconstruction I	Blue Torso and an Angel	22" h x 30" w	Pastel on watercolor paper
51	Reconstruction II	St. Guadaloupe	22" h x 20" w	Acrylic, pastel, and glass on watercolor paper
57	Reconstruction III	Rock Formation (black)	19" h x 25" w	Acrylic, pastel, and glass on pastel paper
58	Reconstruction IV	Rock Formation (blue)	21" h x 27" w	Acrylic, pastel, and glass on pastel paper
79	Reconstruction V	X-Rays (Face)	19" h x 26" w	Acrylic and pastel on pastel paper
54	Reconstruction VI	X-Rays	22" h x 19" w	Acrylic and pastel on pastel paper
46	Reconstruction VII	Diptych	19" h x 34" w	Pastel on watercolor paper
52	Reconstruction VIII	Waterfall	27" h x 21" w	Acrylic, pastel, and glass on pastel paper
64	Reconstruction IX	Woodsy Waterfall	25" h x 19" w	Acrylic, pastel, and glass on pastel paper
63	Reconstruction X	Weathervane	25" h x 19" w	Pastel on pastel paper
89	Reconstruction XI	The Wave	12" h x 19" w	Acrylic and pastel on pastel paper
69	Reconstruction XII	Mink Throw	22" h x 30" w	Pastel on watercolor paper
66	Reconstruction XIII	Lost and Found	22" h x 30" w	Acrylic and pastel on watercolor paper
72	Reconstruction XIV	The Hat	25" h x 20" w	Pastel on pastel paper
76	Reconstruction XV	The Fox and the Bear	29" h x 41" w	Acrylic, pastel, and glass on watercolor paper
86	Reconstruction XVI	Bridge – From Then to Now	19" h x 23" w	Acrylic and pastel on pastel paper
70	Reconstruction XVII	Bridge – From There to Here	19" H x 23" w	Acrylic and pastel on pastel paper
81	Reconstruction XVIII	The Man and the Mantel	25" h x 20" w	Pastel on pastel paper